THE **OFFICIAL** GUIDE TO FOUNDATION LEARNING IN

Hair & Beauty

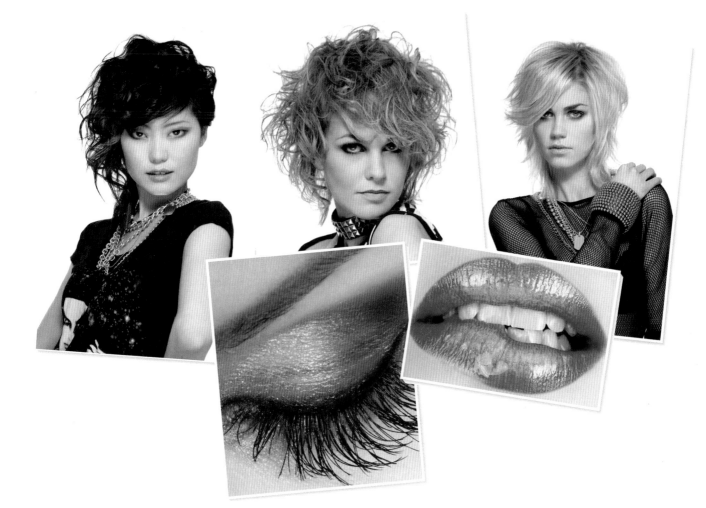

HAIRDRESSING AND BEAUTY INDUSTRY AUTHORITY SERIES

Hairdressing

Student textbooks

Begin Hairdressing: The Official Guide to Level 1 REVISED 2e *Martin Green*

Hairdressing – The Foundations: The Official Guide to Level 2 REVISED 6e *Leo Palladino and Martin Green*

Professional Hairdressing: The Official Guide to Level 3 REVISED 6e *Martin Green and Leo Palladino*

The Official Guide to the City & Guilds Certificate in Salon Service 1e *John Armstrong with Anita Crosland, Martin Green and Lorraine Nordmann*

The Colour Book: The Official Guide to Colour for NVQ Levels 2 and 3 1e *Tracey Lloyd with Christine McMillan-Bodell*

eXtensions: The Official Guide to Hair Extensions 1e *Theresa Bullock*

Salon Management *Martin Green*

Men's Hairdressing: Traditional and Modern Barbering 2e *Maurice Lister*

African-Caribbean Hairdressing 2e *Sandra Gittens*

The World of Hair Colour 1e *John Gray*

The Cutting Book: The Official Guide to Cutting at S/NVQ Levels 2 and 3 *Jane Goldsbro and Elaine White*

Professional Hairdressing titles

Trevor Sorbie: The Bridal Hair Book 1e *Trevor Sorbie and Jacki Wadeson*

The Art of Dressing Long Hair 1 e *Guy Kremer and Jacki Wadeson*

Patrick Cameron: Dressing Long Hair 1e *Patrick Cameron and Jacki Wadeson*

Patrick Cameron: Dressing Long Hair 2 1e *Patrick Cameron and Jacki Wadeson*

Bridal Hair 1e *Pat Dixon and Jacki Wadeson*

Professional Men's Hairdressing: The art of cutting and styling 1e *Guy Kremer and Jacki Wadeson*

Essensuals, The Next Generation Toni and Guy: Step by Step 1e *Sacha Mascolo, Christian Mascolo and Stuart Wesson*

Mahogany Hairdressing: Step to Cutting, Colouring and Finishing Hair 1e *Martin Gannon and Richard Thompson*

Mahogany Hairdressing: Advanced Looks 1e *Martin Gannon and Richard Thompson*

The Total Look: The Style Guide for Hair and Make-up Professional 1e *Ian Mistlin*

Trevor Sorbie: Visions in Hair 1e *Trevor Sorbie, Kris Sorbie and Jacki Wadeson*

The Art of Hair Colouring 1e *David Adams and Jacki Wadeson*

Beauty therapy

Beauty Basics: The Official Guide to Level 1 3e *Lorraine Nordmann*

Beauty Therapy – The Foundations: The Official Guide to Level 2 5e *Lorraine Nordmann*

Professional Beauty Therapy – The Official Guide to Level 3 4e *Lorraine Nordmann*

The Official Guide to the City & Guilds Certificate in Salon Services 1e *John Armstrong with Anita Crosland, Martin Green and Lorraine Nordmann*

The Complete Guide to Make-Up 1e *Suzanne Le Quesne*

The Encyclopedia of Nails 1e *Jacqui Jefford and Anne Swain*

The Art of Nails: A Comprehensive Style Guide to Nail Treatments and Nail Art 1e *Jacqui Jefford*

Nail Artistry 1e *Jacqui Jefford*

The Complete Nail Technician 3e *Marian Newman*

Manicure, Pedicure and Advanced Nail Techniques 1e *Elaine Almond*

The Official Guide to Body Massage 2e *Adele O'Keefe*

An Holistic Guide to Massage 1e *Tina Parsons*

Indian Head Massage 2e *Muriel Burnham-Airey and Adele O'Keefe*

Aromatherapy for the Beauty Therapist 1e *Valerie Worwood*

An Holistic Guide to Reflexology 1e *Tina Parsons*

An Holistic Guide to Anatomy and Physiology 1e *Tina Parsons*

The Essential Guide to Holistic and Complementary Therapy 1e *Helen Beckmann and Suzanne Le Quesne*

The Spa Book 1e *Jane Crebbin-Bailey, Dr John Harcup, and John Harrington*

SPA: The Official Guide to Spa Therapy at Levels 2 and 3, *Joan Scott and Andrea Harrison*

Nutrition: A Practical Approach 1e *Suzanne Le Quesne* Hands on Sports Therapy 1e *Keith Ward*

Encyclopedia of Hair Removal: A Complete Reference to Methods, Techniques and Career Opportunities, *Gill Morris and Janice Brown*

The Anatomy and Physiology Workbook: For Beauty and Holistic Therapies Levels 1–3. *Tina Parsons*

The Anatomy and Physiology CD-Rom

Beautiful Selling: The Complete Guide to Sales Success in the Salon *Ruth Langley*

The Official Guide to the Diploma in Hair and Beauty Studies at Foundation Level 1e *Jane Goldsbro and Elaine White*

The Official Guide to the Diploma in Hair and Beauty Studies at Higher level 1e *Jane Goldsbro and Elaine White*

THE **OFFICIAL** GUIDE TO FOUNDATION LEARNING IN

Hair & Beauty

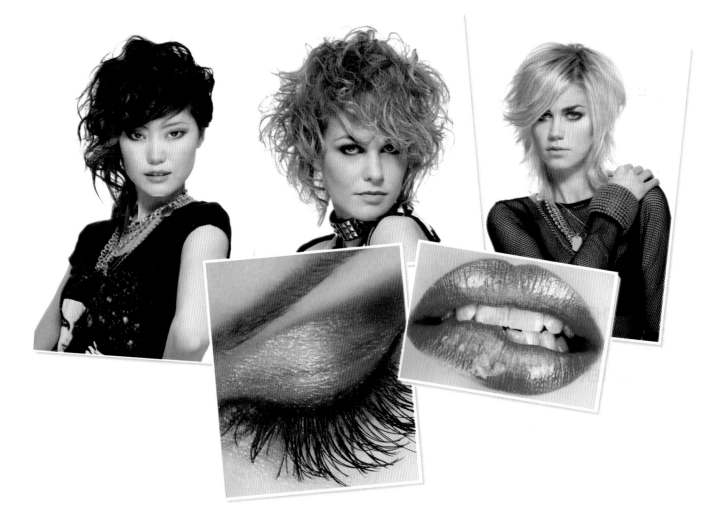

JANE GOLDSBRO AND ELAINE WHITE

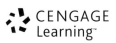

CENGAGE
Learning™

Australia • Brazil • Japan • Korea • Mexico • Singapore • Spain • United Kingdom • United States

CENGAGE
Learning™

The Official Guide to Foundation Learning
in Hair & Beauty
Jane Goldsbro and Elaine White

Publishing Director: Linden Harris
Commissioning Editor: Lucy Mills
Editorial Assistant: Claire Napoli
Project Editor: Lucy Arthy
Production Controller: Eyvett Davis
Marketing Executive: Lauren Redwood
Typesetter: S4 Carlisle, India
Cover design: HCT Creative
Text design: Design Deluxe

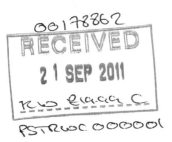
For product information and technology assistance,
contact **emea.info@cengage.com**.
For permission to use material from this text or product,
and for permission queries,
email **clsuk.permissions@cengage.com**.

The Author has asserted the right under the copyright, Designs and Patents Act 1988 to be identified as Author of this book.

British Library Cataloguing-in-Publication Data
A catalogue record for this book is available from the British Library.

ISBN: 978-1-4080-3992-2

Cengage Learning EMEA
Cheriton House, North Way, Andover, Hampshire SP10 5BE
United Kingdom

Cengage Learning products are represented in Canada by
Nelson Education Ltd.

For your lifelong learning solutions, visit
www.cengage.co.uk

Purchase your next print book, e-book or e-chapter at
www.cengagebrain.co.uk

Printed in Malta by Melita Press
1 2 3 4 5 6 7 8 9 10 – 13 12 11

Elaine White

For Oliver, another joy in my life, with love.

Jane Goldsbro

Writing a book is a mixture of frustration, dedication and enjoyment. It takes time to research the content and I'd like to say thanks to all at Cengage Learning for their support.

I'd like to thank my co-author Elaine White; she is a joy to work with and I'm grateful for the time we spend swapping information and ideas. My husband Alan deserves special thanks for his tremendous support and understanding.

As I write the book, Alan takes on the household chores whilst I bounce ideas off him, make him listen to my text and he plots the crosswords and wordsearches on his computer. Something my mother did by hand on my very first book. Thanks Mum.

Contents

About the authors

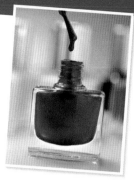

Jane Goldsbro

A qualified hairdresser since 1982, Jane is one of the most influential educators in hair and beauty today. Her skills in developing the structure of UK hair and beauty education are renowned throughout the world.

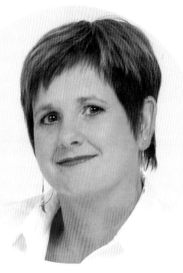

Jane's early career as a hairdresser took her through a formative path where she ran salons and worked for some of the best companies and key influencers in the field of education such as Alan International, and Redken where she worked as one of their top technicians.

At an early stage of her career, Jane was a regional winner of the L'Oréal Colour Trophy at the tender age of 17 while still training at North Lindsey College. This led her to start a teaching career at North Lindsey. However, the deep-rooted commitment to continue learning saw Jane taking on her biggest challenge when she went to work at Habia.

1992 saw Jane start at Habia as Development Manager for Hairdressing and within four years she had risen to Director of Standards and Qualifications. This role saw her take on bigger challenges each and every year. Not only did Jane enhance the development of hairdressing education, she began to expand Habia's remit into beauty therapy. Since those heady days of endless development meetings, running standards workshops and training international educators in Habia techniques, Jane still found time to develop her skills.

An established writer of technical material for Habia, Jane is also the author of two hairdressing study guides and four hairdressing text books including *The Official Guides to the Diploma in Hair and Beauty Studies* for both the Foundation and Higher Levels, on behalf of Cengage Learning, the leading publisher in hair and beauty. Her expertise in training and assessing has enabled her to work with and support all the hair and beauty awarding organizations in the UK in the development of qualifications. At the inception of a new regulatory regime by the UK government in training, Jane became one of the first inspectors for the Adult Learning Inspectorate that is now part of Ofsted.

Her role at Habia as Director of Standards and Qualifications now covers all six sectors of Habia's portfolio in hair, beauty, nails, spa, barbering and African-type hair. She is responsible for setting the standard for hair and beauty education from schools to university graduates in the UK and with our international partners in Spain, Italy, Japan, China, Malta, India, Syria and the USA.

Truly one of the most knowledgeable hair and beauty educators in the world.

Elaine White

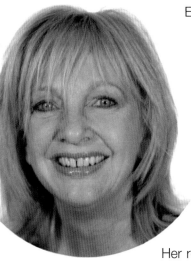

Elaine White has a lifetime of experience in the hair and beauty sector. She has been involved with the development and implementation of some of the most influential hair and beauty programmes in colleges, schools and in work based learning.

Throughout her career, Elaine has been involved in researching the processes and developing systems that have raised standards in the hair and beauty sector. She has contributed massively to hair and beauty education, the standards for which are renowned throughout the world. Her passion for learning and development has taken her from the hair and beauty industry into the challenging world of further and higher education. Here she has spent more than 16 years as an educator before joining Habia, the Standard Setting Body for the hair and beauty sector.

Her role with Habia allowed Elaine to work with a diverse range of stakeholders from schools and colleges to learning providers and universities to develop and introduce innovative learning programmes, apprenticeships and foundation degrees. One of her most rewarding projects was to research the incidence of dyslexia in the hairdressing industry. This project culminated in presenting the findings to an invited audience at the House of Lords, the home of the upper chamber the UK parliament.

Elaine continues to provide support and expertise to schools and colleges as a technical author, educational consultant, moderator and examiner for hair and beauty qualifications.

If this wasn't enough, Elaine is also an additional inspector for Ofsted. Her passion for quality is paramount and clearly evident through her work.

Acknowledgements

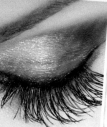

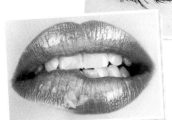

Jane Goldsbro and Elaine White would like to thank Lucy Mills, Claire Napoli and Lucy Arthy for their support and guidance during the writing of the book. Their thanks also go to Alan Goldsbro and Graham White for all their valuable help.

The authors and the publishers would like to thank the following:

For their help with the photo shoot:
Make up: Louise Young (Habia Skills Team)
Photography: Ed Cartledge from Sort to Films Ltd
Model agency: DK Model Management
Models: Jessica Renton
       Glen Wood
       Chloe

For providing pictures for the book:
Habia and Habia Skills Team
Saks
Dr John Gray
i-stock photography
L'Oréal Professional
Goldwell
Namast
Alamy
REM
Shortcuts
Shutterstock.com
Digitalskillet
DR H.M Becks
Guinot
Paiadara
Beauty Express
Dr A.L Wright
Wellcome photo library
Dino
Ellisons
Star Nails
Salon Systems
Millenium Nails
Sorisa
Hobbs Salon, Temple Fortune, London
Kiss and Make-up
Majestic Towels Ltd
Screenface Ltd
Louise Young Cosmetics
The Color Wheel Company
Antica Erboristeria srl

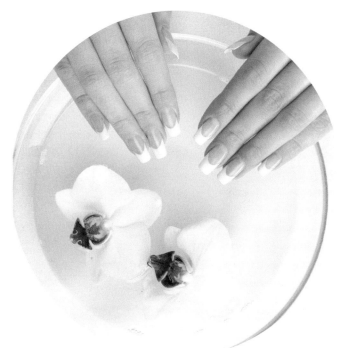

Foreword

I am delighted that two people whom I have known and worked with for a long time have again joined forces to write this fantastic book.

Jane Goldsbro and Elaine White are also co-authors of *The Cutting Book: The Official Guide to Cutting for S/NVQ Levels 2 and 3* and *The Official Guide to the Diploma in Hair and Beauty Studies at Foundation and Higher Level*. They are authorities in their field and their input into the hairdressing industry is immense. Through their work with Habia they push forward the standards for hair and beauty education worldwide.

Elaine has over 30 years' experience within the industry, spending eight years with Habia as Senior Development Manager and over 15 years as a hairdressing lecturer and course team leader. Elaine is a true professional whose exacting standards and dedication to her work have enabled her to focus on the end product with outstanding results. At Habia, Elaine was responsible for Apprenticeships and Foundation Degree Frameworks.

Jane has almost 30 years' experience within the hairdressing industry, including salon management, educator and for the last 11 years as Director of Standards and Qualifications at Habia. The commitment she has to her work is phenomenal. From writing standards, managing people and relationships with partners to international development, her wide vision means that she has an impressive ability to see the steps needed to achieve an end result. Jane's contribution to the hair and beauty curriculum has impacted throughout the world; as a developer of structured education she is very much in demand across all continents where her views are consistently sought.

The Foundation Learning programme in Hair and Beauty has been developed to offer a more flexible and personalized approach to studies and the combination of classroom learning with practical hands-on experience prepares young people for employment and further training. As well as broadening the options available to young people, the Foundation Learning programme also brings a range of benefits to employers by providing an overall framework to easily identify key skills of new recruits. The Foundation Learning programmes are being implemented nationally between 2010 and 2013.

Alan Goldsbro
Chief Executive Officer
Habia
2011

About the book

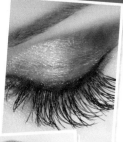

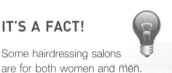

ACTIVITY

Find out which services are offered in your local salons. Make a visit or look on their websites.

Activity boxes feature within all chapters and provide additional tasks for you to further your understanding

IT'S A FACT!

Some hairdressing salons are for both women and men. They are known as 'unisex' salons.

It's A Fact! boxes draw your attention to interesting facts and information about the hair and beauty industries

SIGNPOST PLTS

PLTS

Independent enquirer

PLTS signposts show where your six personal learning and thinking skills can be developed by using the activities suggested

WWW
WEB LINK

www.hji.co.uk Go to this link to find out more about some of the fantastic looks that are created by top hairdressers.

Weblinks suggest useful websites and other online sources for further research and additional information about the industries

WHAT'S NEXT?

Once you have completed your basic training for African type hair, you could specialize in braiding or hair extensions.

What's Next? boxes appear throughout the book and indicate what the next stage of learning is for a particular topic

TOP TIP

If your client has oily hair, apply the conditioner only to the ends of the hair.

Top Tips share the authors' experiences and provide positive suggestions to improve knowledge and skills

SIGNPOST PSD

PSD

Preparation for work

As part of your personal and social development you have to prepare yourself for work. You need to find out about job roles.

PSD signposts show where activities and tasks can improve your personal and social development

SIGNPOST ERR

ERR

As part of employment rights and responsibilities when working in a salon you will need to have a basic knowledge on issues relating to your employment terms and conditions and disciplinary procedures.

ERR signposts appear in core chapters and show where particular topics connect to employability skills required in the hair and beauty sector

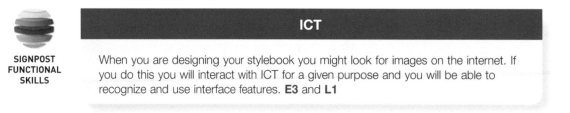

ICT

When you are designing your stylebook you might look for images on the internet. If you do this you will interact with ICT for a given purpose and you will be able to recognize and use interface features. **E3** and **L1**

SIGNPOST FUNCTIONAL SKILLS

Functional Skills show where your information communication technologies (ICT), Maths, and English skills can be developed by using the activities suggested

Carrying out a hand massage

Step-by-step method for a hand massage procedure

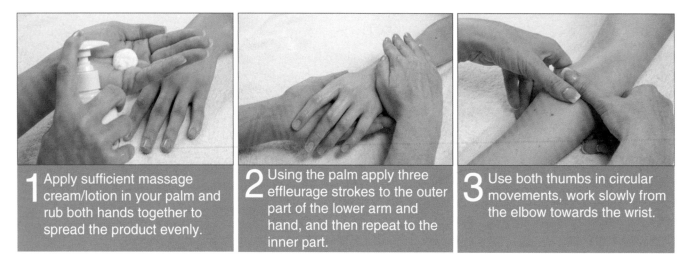

1 Apply sufficient massage cream/lotion in your palm and rub both hands together to spread the product evenly.

2 Using the palm apply three effleurage strokes to the outer part of the lower arm and hand, and then repeat to the inner part.

3 Use both thumbs in circular movements, work slowly from the elbow towards the wrist.

Step-by-step sequences demonstrate the featured practical skills using colour photographs to enhance understanding

ASSESSMENT ACTIVITIES

Activity 1 E1 – L1

How do you do that?

Look at the following hairstyles and then read the list of hairstyling techniques. Match the technique you would use to achieve the hairstyles.

Assessment Activities are provided at the end of each chapter. You can use the questions to prepare for oral and written assessments and help test your knowledge throughout. Seek guidance from your supervisor/assessor if there are areas you are unsure of

About the Website

Find activity answers and extra puzzles online

Check your answers to all of the assessment activity questions in this book and find printable crosswords and wordsearches for you to try by visiting:

www.cengage.co.uk/goldsbro_white

- Answers to all end-of-chapter assessment activities
- Crosswords to accompany each chapter
- Wordsearches to accompany each chapter
- Solutions to all crosswords and wordsearches

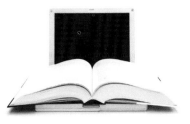

Crossword E3–L1

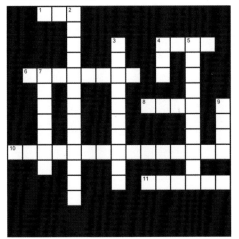

Across

1 This is known as a work-ready qualification (3)

4 These can be found in exotic locations (4)

6 A nail technician will carry out this treatment on the hands and nails (8)

8 A freelance hairdresser might visit their clients here (4)

10 This person is likely to carry out a waxing treatment (two words 6,9)

11 A beauty therapy is likely to apply this (two words 4,2)

Down

2 You will receive this if you successfully complete a training programme (13)

3 The workplace of a barber (2 words 6,4)

4 The number of industries in the hair and beauty sector (3)

5 This person is paid to train while they are employed in a salon or spa (10)

7 Relaxing is carried out on this type of hair (7)

9 A pedicure is carried out on these (4)

Wordsearch E1–L1

Hidden in the grid below are 32 words. Can you find them all?

APPRENTICE	HAIRDRESSERS	SALON
ASSESSOR	HAIRDRESSING	SECTOR
BARBERING	INDUSTRY	SHAVING
BEAUTY	JOB	SPA
CAREER	LEARNING	STYLING
COLLEGE	LECTURER	STYLIST
COLOURING	MANICURE	TEACHER
COMMISSION	NAILS	TECHNICIANS
CUTTING	PEDICURE	THERAPISTS
EMPLOYED	PERMING	WAXING
FREELANCE	SALARY	

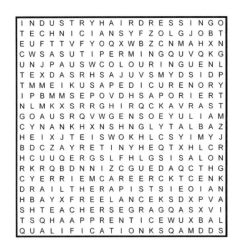

```
I N D U S T R Y H A I R D R E S S I N G O
T E C H N I C I A N S Y F Z O L G J O B T
E U F T T V F Y O Q X W B Z C N M A H X N
C W S A S U T I P E R M I N G Q U V Q K G
U N J P A U S W C O L O U R I N G U E N L
T E X D A S R H S A J U V S M Y D S I D P
T M M E I K U S A P E D I C U R E N O R Y
I P B M M S E P O V D H S A P O R I E R T
N L M K X S R R G H I R Q C K A V R A S T
G O A U S R Q V W G E N S O E Y U L I A M
C Y N A N K H X N S H N G L Y T A L B A Z
H E I X J T E I S W O K H L C S Y I M Y J
B D C Z A Y R E T I N Y H E Q T X H L C R
H C U U Q E R G S L F H L G S I S A L O N
R K R Q B D N N I Z C G U E D A Q C T H G
C Y E R R I E M C A R E E R C K T C E N K
D R A I L T H E R A P I S T S I E O I A N
H B A Y X F R E E L A N C E K S D X P V A
S H T E A C H E R S E G R A G Q A S X V I
T S Q H A A P P R E N T I C E W U X B A L
Q U A L I F I C A T I O N K S Q A M D D S
```

Foundation Learning programme

Introduction

Foundation Learning (FL) is the national suite of learning for 14–19-year-olds and adult learners. An individual learning programme is agreed to reflect both the learner's entry point and intended destination to other training programmes, independent living or employment. The stepping-stones of Foundation Learning are captured in different qualifications that are on the Qualification Credit Framework. These qualifications provide flexibility to capture different themes and levels of learning. All Awarding Organizations offering these qualifications within the hair and beauty sector will use the same unit contents but may assess them differently and put them into different qualifications such as Awards, Certificates or Diplomas at Entry Level or Level 1:

- An Award is the smallest type of qualification of 1–10 credits.
- A Certificate is a medium sized qualification with 11–36 credits.
- A Diploma is the largest type of qualification with 37+ credits.

The Foundation Learning programme

A Foundation Learning programme is flexible and designed to meet the needs of individual learners.

The Foundation Learning programme will include:

- Vocational learning.
- Functional skills.
- Personal and social development learning.

Learners on a Foundation Learning programme might include those:

- In mainstream education working at Entry Level and Level 1.
- On key stage 4 engagement programmes.
- On entry to employment programmes.
- With special educational needs.
- With learning difficulties and/or disabilities.
- Not in education, employment or training (NEET).
- Attending pupil referral units.

Overview of the Foundation Learning programme

As part of the programme young people and adults will be assessed to find out the level at which they are able to learn most effectively. Learners will also receive ongoing reviews to identify the support required to ensure they achieve their learning goals. Initial advice and guidance will be provided throughout the Foundation Learning programme to support access to services such as carer, child care, financial and housing advice.

Initial assessment ⟶ Personalized learning programme: ⟶ progression destination

- Vocational /subject-based learning (8–40 Credits)
- Personal and social development learning (3–21 Credits)
- Functional skills (15 Credits)

⟵———————————————————————————⟶
Information advice and guidance

Foundation Learning programmes for hair and beauty

Typically a Foundation Learning programme for someone interested in hair and beauty will include:

A vocational qualification in hair and beauty covering topics such as skincare and make-up, nail art, hair care and styling, health and safety and understanding the hair and beauty industries.

A personal and social development qualification covering topics such as working towards goals, preparing for work, healthy living, individual rights and responsibilities and managing own money.

Functional skills in English, mathematics and information communication technology at a level that is appropriate for the learner.

Progression from a Foundation Learning programme

The Foundation Learning programme will support progression into a range of different destinations.

Progression can be into:

Diplomas	Apprenticeships	GCSEs	Full Level 2
Employment	Supported employment	Living more independently	Other 14–19 qualifications

Progression from a Foundation Learning programme in hair and beauty

There are many progression routes available for learners following the Foundation Learning programme in hair and beauty. Destinations would include:

Apprenticeships (employed or programme led) completing a job ready qualification such as a National Vocational Qualification (NVQ)

- Hairdressing.
- Barbering.
- Beauty therapy.
- Nail services.

College or school-based programmes completing preparation for work qualifications such as a Vocational Qualification (VQ) from Levels 1 to 3

- Hairdressing.
- Barbering.
- Beauty therapy.
- Nail services.

Diploma in Hair and Beauty Studies completed in partnerships of school, colleges and learning providers

- Diploma in Hair and Beauty Studies at Foundation Level.
- Diploma in Hair and Beauty Studies at Higher Level.
- Diploma in Hair and Beauty Studies at Advanced Level.

1
Introduction to the hair and beauty sector

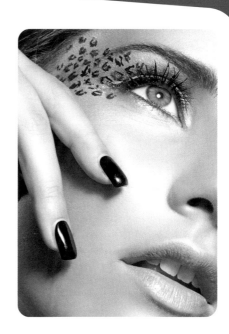

> "The best career advice given to the young is:
> 'Find out what you like doing best and get someone to pay you for doing it.'
>
> KATHERINE DUNHAM, AMERICAN DANCER 1909–2006

In this chapter you are going to learn about:

- Job roles in the hair and beauty sector.
- The different types of salon for the six different industries and the services they offer.
- Working patterns in the hair and beauty sector.
- Pay structure for the hair and beauty sector.
- Learning programmes in hair and beauty.
- Employment rights and responsibilities in the hair and beauty sector.
- The career opportunities that will be open to you.
- Where you can find more information about careers.

Introduction

Can you think of a better job than one where, as you are working, you can be cruising in the Caribbean or working on the set of the latest, block-busting movie? Or, you could be your own boss – as young as the age of 20. You can do all these if you train to work in any of the hair and beauty sectors. Of course, the very top jobs are hard to get, and everyone has to start at the bottom and work their way up. Working in the hair and beauty sector is not an easy option. You have to work hard and be creative and determined if you want to succeed. But, the work is very rewarding. On a recent investigation about people who are happy in their jobs, hairdressers and beauty therapists topped the 'happiness' scale.

IT'S A FACT!

The term **sector** is the one general term that is used to describe all the separate industries found in hair and beauty.

IT'S A FACT!

Some hairdressing salons are for both women and men. They are known as 'unisex' salons.

ACTIVITY

Find out which services are offered in your local salons. Make a visit or look on their websites.

SIGNPOST PLTS

PLTS

Independent enquirer

WWW

WEB LINK

www.hji.co.uk Go to this link to find out more about some of the fantastic looks that are created by top hairdressers.

WHAT'S NEXT?

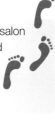

After training to work in a salon as a hairdresser you could do more training to become a teacher of hairdressing.

ACTIVITY

Find out which services are offered in your local barber shops. Make a visit or look on their websites.

SIGNPOST PLTS

PLTS

Independent enquirer

Job roles in the hair and beauty sector

You may think you know what the job roles are in the hair and beauty sector. You see people working in salons. But there are many other jobs that people who work in the hair and beauty sector do that you may not be aware of.

Six industries of the sector

There are six industries in the hair and beauty sector. They are:

- Hairdressing.
- Barbering.
- African-Caribbean hairdressing and barbering.
- Beauty therapy.
- Nail services.
- Spa therapy.

Hairdressing If you work as a hairdresser you will provide services for the hair and scalp. Hairdressers offer many different services which include:

- Styling: setting, dressing and blow drying hair.
- Colouring: highlighting and using permanent and semi-permanent colours.
- Cutting: creating amazing looks using different cutting techniques.

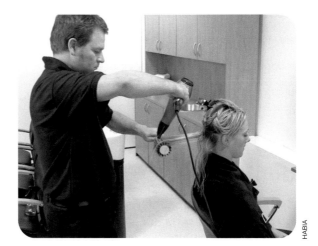

Hairdressing salon and hairdresser working on a client

Barbering If you work as a barber you will provide treatments and services for the hair and scalp for men and boys. Barbers offer many different services which include:

- Cutting: creating a range of looks, traditional and modern, using different cutting techniques.

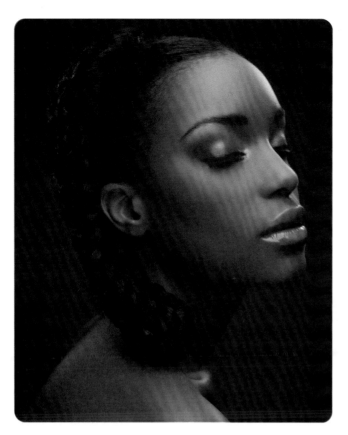

You can learn how to create braids and twists like this if you complete a qualification for African type hairdressing

WEB LINK

Many barber shops have a blue, red and white striped pole outside. Look at these websites to find out why: http://www.barberpole.com or http://www.thamessalon.com/site/barberhistory.htm. You can also read about the history of barbering.

IT'S A FACT!

The word barber comes from the Latin word *barba*, which means beard.

- Shaving and facial hair trimming: removing facial hair or cutting the facial hair into different shapes.

- Colouring: highlighting and using permanent and semi-permanent colours.

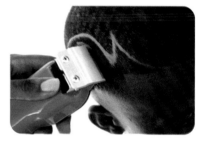

Cutting patterns into hair

African-Caribbean hairdressing and barbering   There are salons that specialize in providing services for clients with African type hair. You can read more about African type hair in Chapter 7, 'Hair care'. The services carried out in African type hair salons will be similar to those seen in any hairdressing salon, but you will also see other services such as:

- Relaxing: where the natural curl of the hair is straightened.

- Cutting hair into 3D patterns: sometimes known as hair tattooing.

- Twisting: styling natural African type hair by twisting into styles such as bantu knots.

- Thermal styling: styling hair using a variety of heated equipment.

Beauty therapy   If you work in a beauty therapy salon you will provide treatments for the face and body. Beauty therapists offer many different treatments which include:

- Face massage: improving the appearance and condition of the skin.

- Waxing: removing hair using waxing techniques.

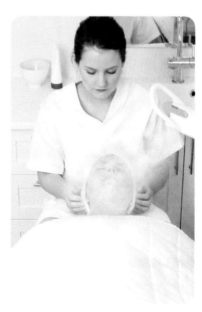

A beauty therapist working on a client

A nail technician working on a client

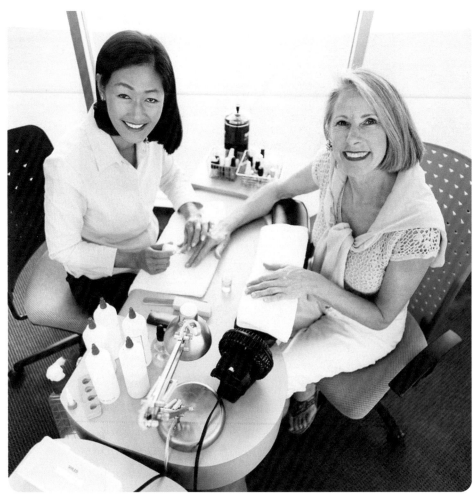

WHAT'S NEXT?

After training to become a barber in a barber's shop, you could work as a freelance barber. This means that you do not have your own salon, but travel around to cut the hair of men and boys in their own homes, or in hospitals or care homes.

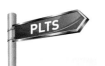

ACTIVITY

Find out which services are offered in your local African type hair salon. Make a visit or look on their websites.

SIGNPOST PLTS

Independent enquirer

WHAT'S NEXT?

Once you have completed your basic training for African type hair, you could specialize in braiding or hair extensions.

WWW

WEB LINK

Look at this web link for hairstyling from Black Hair and Beauty magazine: **http://www .blackbeautyandhair.com/ html/channels/hairgallery.asp**. There are lots of other areas you can look at, such as make-up and nail care.

- Providing eyelash and eyebrow treatments: lash extensions and lash and brow tinting.
- Make-up: making up clients for day, evening and special occasions.

Nail services If you work in a nail salon you will provide treatments for the hands and feet. Nail technicians offer many different treatments which include:

- Manicure and pedicure: improving the appearance of the nails and skin on the hands and feet.
- Nail art: creating patterns and designs on the nails.
- Extending nails: making nails look longer and stronger.

Spa therapy If you work in a spa you will provide treatments for the body and mind. Spa therapists offer many different treatments which include:

- Water treatments: flotation, steam and sauna.
- Indian head massage: massaging the head to create a sense of well-being.
- Massage using aromatherapy oils: a body massage to create a feeling of relaxation.

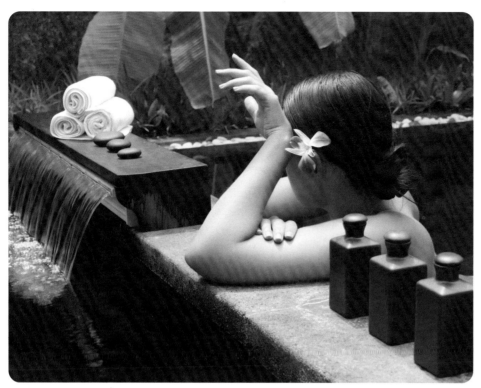

Spas can be found in exotic locations all around the world

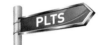

ACTIVITY

Find out which treatments are offered in your local beauty therapy salons. Make a visit or look on their websites.

SIGNPOST
PLTS

Independent enquirer

ACTIVITY

If you go on a work placement to a hair or beauty salon, ask permission to take some photographs of the different hair and beauty treatments and services taking place. Write a review about your work placement and include the images you have taken.

SIGNPOST
PLTS

Creative thinker
Independent enquirer
Reflective learner

ICT
When you write your review you can use software to:
E3 and L1 format and edit your work and to insert images.

SIGNPOST
FUNCTIONAL
SKILL

The different types of salon for the six different industries

When you walk down your own high street you will see that there are lots of different types of hair and beauty salon.

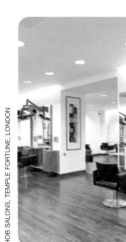

HOB SALONS, TEMPLE FORTUNE, LONDON

A typical, modern hairdressing salon

Hairdressing salon

The majority of hairdressing salons are open plan. This means that you can see all the stylists and all the clients in one large room.

Some hairdressing salons can be very noisy places as they play loud music; others have a calm and relaxing atmosphere. The look and atmosphere of the hairdressing salon is designed and planned to meet the needs of the majority of clients whom the salon owner wishes to attract. Some salon designs are modern and some have a more traditional look. Some are decorated with very bright colours, and others are neutral. Some salons may have other treatment rooms for beauty or nail services.

Barber shop

Many barber shops can look very different to hairdressing salons. Barber shops often have a very traditional look, which many men prefer. The decoration is often designed to look more masculine.

African-Caribbean hairdressing and barbering

A business that specializes in African type hair may not look any different to other types of hairdressing salon and barber shop. However, there are some salons that like to re-create African-Caribbean culture, so these may have a much more laid back atmosphere.

Beauty therapy salon

The environment of a beauty therapy salon is usually very calming and peaceful. Some beauty salons can look very clinical, while others are decorated in neutral tones with softly lit treatment rooms to aid relaxation during massage. Any music played is likely to be soothing and relaxing.

WHAT'S NEXT?

Some beauty therapists take additional training and qualifications to become an expert in the application of semi-permanent make-up.

IT'S A FACT!

Make-up is not just for women. Male make-up ranges are becoming more popular. Have a look at this website **http://www .astonmitchell.co.uk/**

ACTIVITY

Find out which treatments are offered in your local nail salons. Make a visit or look on their websites.

SIGNPOST PLTS

Independent enquirer

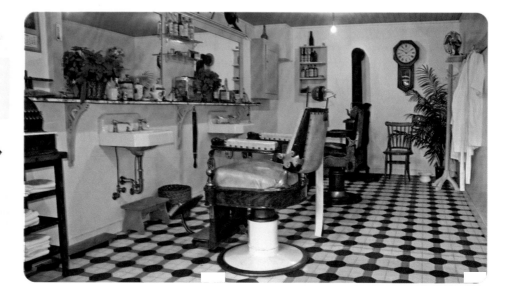

A traditional barber shop

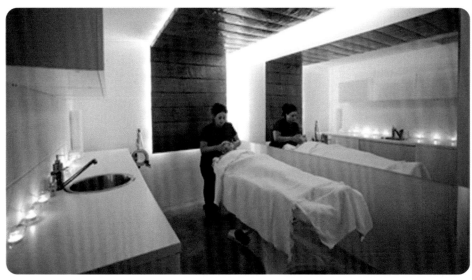

COURTESY OF WWW.KISSANDMAKEUP.TV

Beauty treatment rooms are softly lit to relax the client

WEB LINK

Look at this link about nail art – you can see how to create the designs. **http://www .salongeek.com/nail-art- tutorials/**

Nail salon

A nail salon is likely to be open plan and brightly lit. Many spas, beauty therapy salons or hairdressing salons will have a 'nail bar'. This is an area of the salon that is set aside for hand and feet treatments and services.

WHAT'S NEXT?

Once you have gained some experience working in a nail salon, you could open your own business.

Spa

Spas can vary from a day spa in the middle of a town, to residential spas in a beautiful, rural location. You can also find spas in very exotic locations all over the world. Within a spa you are likely to find most, if not all, the industries in the hair and beauty sector. At a spa you may be able to have your hair styled and receive a beauty therapy and nail service. Spas will be restful, relaxing places, with soft, soothing music. In large spas you will find lots of individual treatments rooms and large open areas with different types of pool and water treatment.

ACTIVITY

Find out which treatments are offered in your local spas. Make a visit or look on their websites.

SIGNPOST PLTS

Independent enquirer

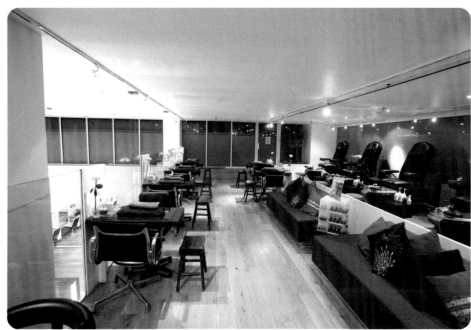

URBAN RETREAT AT HARRODS, KNIGHTSBRIDGE, LONDON

WEB LINK

Have a look at this web link and play a game to make a successful spa **http://www .gamesgames.com/game/ Beauty-Resort.html** You have to keep your clients happy, or you will lose them. The game will also develop your time management skills.

Nail salon

WHAT'S NEXT?

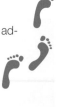

Some spa therapists take additional qualifications to provide treatments for alternative therapies such as Reiki, stone therapy or reflexology.

ACTIVITY

Choose one of the hair and beauty sectors and then create a display showing the different treatments and services that you can have. Find some pictures to put in your display of clients showing the '*before*' and '*after*' for the services. The display could be used at a careers event. You could present your mood boards and talk to others about career opportunities in the hair and beauty sector.

SIGNPOST PLTS

Self-manager
Creative thinker
Independent enquirer

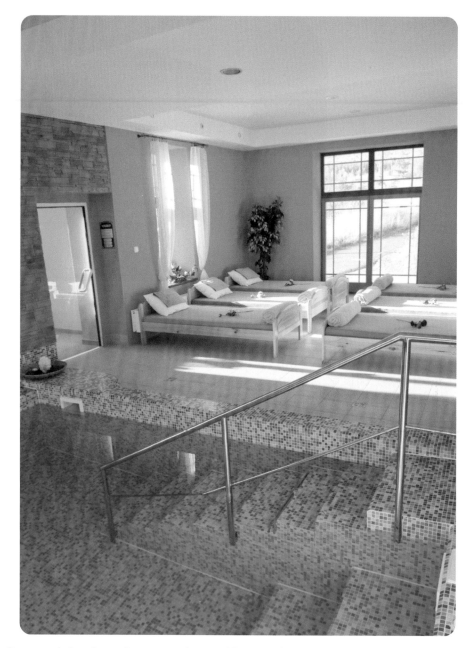

Spas are relaxing places where you can have a wide range of treatments and services

SIGNPOST FUNCTIONAL SKILL

English

When you talk to others about careers in the hair and beauty sector you will be able to show you can:

E3 use appropriate language in a formal discussion

L1 present information clearly and in an appropriate language.

Working patterns in the hair and beauty sector

Do you want a job where you begin work at 9.00am every morning, finish work at 5.00pm every evening and have Saturdays off? If you do, then working in the hair and beauty sector is probably not for you. Some salons may open and close at these times, but most will have late nights and all will open on Saturdays and even Sundays. If you work in a spa you may have to work in shifts. Many spas are linked to hotels or other leisure businesses. This means they are open for seven days each week from early in the morning until very late at night.

Pay structure in the hair and beauty sector

Some people think that if you work in any of the hair and beauty sectors, you will not earn very much money. But this can be said about many jobs, especially while you are training. When you first start work, you will not be able to do very much, so your pay will be limited. As you progress through your qualifications and are able to do more, your pay will increase. Today the average salary across the hair and beauty sector is £229 per week. This means that some people earn less than this – and some earn more.

Happiness table – City & Guilds

Position	Profession	Position	Profession
1	Beauticians	9 =	Engineers
2 =	Hairdressers	9 =	Architects
2 =	Armed forces	13 =	Journalists
4	Catering/chefs	13 =	Mechanics/automotive
5	Retail staff	13 =	Human resources
6 =	Teachers	16	Call centre
6 =	Marketing/PR2	17 =	IT specialists
6 =	Accountants	17 =	Nurses
9 =	Secretaries/receptionists	17 =	Banker/finance
9 =	Plumbers	17 =	Builders/construction

WWW
WEB LINK
Look at this website to find out more about the jobs available in the beauty therapy industry: http://www.hji.co.uk/jobs/browse/beauty.htm

IT'S A FACT!
Some very exclusive salons have special rooms that are more private for VIP clients.

IT'S A FACT!
People with African type hair are from all races.

IT'S A FACT!
Some salons specialize in natural African type hair, while others also carry out services on chemically treated African type hair.

WWW
WEB LINK
You can look at lots of different types of salons for the hair, beauty and spa industries by checking out this website: http://www.saloninteriordesign.co.uk/

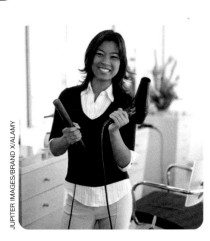

JUPITER IMAGES/BRAND X/ALAMY

A happy hairdresser

SIGNPOST
FUNCTIONAL
SKILL

ACTIVITY

Design your own hairdressing sa-lon, beauty therapy salon, barber shop, nail salon or spa. Use paper with squares marked, such as graph paper, so that one square represents one metre. How big will you make your salon? Decide where you would place your salon furniture. Choose a colour scheme for you salon or spa. Will you make it bright or neutral? Look at the website in the web link on page 9 to get some ideas.

SIGNPOST PLTS

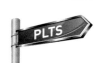

Independent enquirer

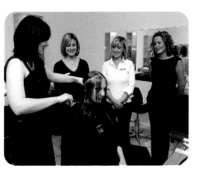

IMAGE COURTESY OF SAKS, WWW.SAKS.CO.UK

Students in a hairdressing class

Many employers pay their staff **commission**. This is a percentage of the money paid by clients for the treatments and services that are carried out that is given to the stylist or therapist as part of their wage. So, the more clients you have and the busier you are, the more commission you will get and the more you will earn.

Although you need to earn money, job satisfaction is also very important.

If you work hard and study for more qualifications you can earn high salaries in the hair and beauty sector. For example, managers and teachers in hair and beauty will be paid at the same level as other managers and teachers.

You can also be self-employed or own your own salon. Then, your salary will reflect the success and profitability of your own business.

Mathematics

When you plan your salon you will be making a scale drawing. Calculate how big the floor would be in real life. Many salons have tiled floors. Find out how many tiles you would need to cover the floor area. When you do this you will:

E3   use metric units in everyday situations and complete simple calculations involving measure

L1   solve problems requiring calculation with common measures

SIGNPOST PSD

PSD

Managing money

When you work in the hair and beauty sector you will take payments from clients. You need to be good at dealing with money. You can play 'Check Out Challenge' game to see how quickly you can work out the change required for the customers: **http://www.bgfl.org/bgfl/custom/resources_ftp/client_ftp/ks2/maths/ shop_counter/index.htm**
When you begin work you will receive a wage. The amount you are paid is recorded on a **pay slip**. Play this 'Payslip Puzzler' game to learn about the other information found on a pay slip: **http://www.mymoneyonline.org/Fortunity/Game/launchPayslip.aspx**

Learning programmes for hair and beauty

If you decide that you would like to work in the hair and beauty sector, you must determine which type of programme you will study. You can follow a college or school-based programme. Or when you are 16, if you feel you are ready to be employed, you can become an apprentice.

College or school-based programmes for hair and beauty

You can study for a National Vocational Qualification (NVQ) or a Vocation Quali-fication (VQ) from Levels 1–3 in a college of further education or in some schools. During your time on the learning programme you will spend some time with an employer on work placement. This gives you a true picture of what a commercial salon or spa is like.

Apprenticeships in the hair and beauty sector

If you decide to become an apprentice, you will be employed in a salon or spa. You will receive a wage while you study for your qualifications. You will complete an **apprenticeship framework**. An apprenticeship framework is a collection of individual qualifications and when you complete them all, you will receive an **apprenticeship** certificate. The certificate will show others that you gained you qualifications by working in a salon through **work-based learning**.

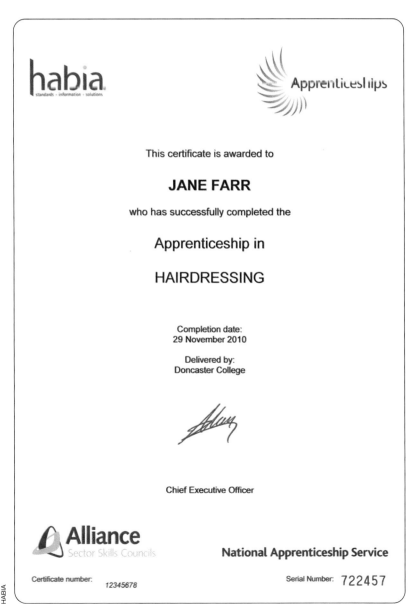

An apprenticeship certificate is awarded when you complete the apprenticeship

ACTIVITY

Look at the opening times of the salons in your area. How many of them have a late night? What time do they close? Discuss with other members of your class why salons are open late on some evenings each week.

SIGNPOST PLTS

Creative thinker

IT'S A FACT!

The survey to find the happiest workers was carried out by City & Guilds. Hairdressers were at the top of the scale and secretarial, banking, insurance and finance workers were the least happy in their work.

IT'S A FACT!

To be successful in salon ownership, you need to develop management skills as well as technical skills. You can go to university and study for a degree in salon management.

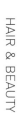

WEB LINK

Check out the following websites for jobs in the hair and beauty industries: **www.hji.co.uk/jobs/** and **www.hairandbeautyjobs .com**

To complete the apprenticeship certificate you must complete:

- **NVQ**: this is the qualification for the industry you have chosen to work in.
- **Functional skills** in English and Maths and sometimes information communication technology (ICT): these are the skills you need for work and everyday living.
- **Employment rights and responsibilities**: this is information you will need to ensure that you are aware of your rights and responsibilities in the workplace.

SIGNPOST FUNCTIONAL SKILL

English
When you study newspapers or magazines for jobs and salaries you will:
E3 read and understand the purpose and content of straightforward texts to understand the main points
L1 read and understand the purpose and content of straightforward texts to utilize information contained in the texts.

ACTIVITY

Look at job advertisements for the hair and beauty sector. See how much salary is offered.

SIGNPOST PLTS

Independent Enquirer

IT'S A FACT!

An NVQ is known as a **work-ready qualification**. A VQ, which can also include the Diploma in Hair and Beauty Studies, is a **preparation for work qualification**.

WHAT'S NEXT?

As an apprentice you will learn about your employment rights and responsibilities.

More about employment rights and responsibilities (ERR)

All apprentices are employed. Because of this they need to know what their rights and responsibilities are in the workplace. They also need to know the rights and responsibilities of their employer.

You will learn about:

- **Equal rights for recruitment**: how the interview process should be fair so you are not discriminated against.
- **Equal rights in employment**: the right to have a **contract of employment**.
- **The working time directive and minimum wage**: the numbers of hours you should be working each week, and the right to have the correct wage for the job you are doing.
- **Health and safety**: so you can work safely in a healthy environment.
- **Career pathways and industry structure**: you will learn about the ways you can progress in the hair and beauty sector, and important organizations that can help and support you.
- **The grievance and disciplinary procedure**: how you can tell your employer about a complaint and the right for an employer to discipline staff following fair procedures.
- **Issues of public concern**: how customers are now more aware of their rights and good practices such as client care, qualified staff and care for the environment.

SIGNPOST PSD

Environmental awareness and individual rights and responsibilities

If you are an apprentice in the hair and beauty sector you will learn your rights and responsibilities in employment. Your personal and social development unit about Individual rights and responsibilities is about your individual rights and responsibilities in society. One part of the employment rights and responsibilities unit regarding Issues of public concern is about looking after the environment. This is similar to the content of your personal and social development unit on environmental awareness.

WEB LINK

You can find out more about your employment rights and responsibilities by looking at this web link: http://www.habia.org/uploads/ERR%20course%20guidelines.pdf

Career opportunities and progression in the hair and beauty sector

Training to work in any of the hair and beauty sectors is not easy. The skills have to be learned over a long period of time. And, you can never say that you know how to do everything. You have to keep training for the rest of your working life. You will never know it all. But this makes the job really interesting.

Everyone who works in the hair and beauty sectors will have to start at the bottom and work their way up. The level you choose to work at is down to you. Many people are very happy to work in salons once they have completed their basic training. Some like to move into other areas of the hair and beauty sectors, such as teaching and training, or sales and marketing.

Have a look at the career progression table to see which job may be open to you.

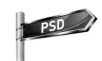

SIGNPOST PSD

Preparation for work

As part of your personal and social development you have to prepare yourself for work. You need to find out about job roles. Look at the career progression table on page 14 and see if there are any job roles that you might like to find out more about.

SIGNPOST PSD

Preparation for work

As part of your personal and social development you have to prepare yourself for work. You need to know the skills and qualities that are required by employers. Complete the next activity about employability skills and see if you have the right skills for the hair and beauty sectors.

ACTIVITY

There are certain skills that employers like to see. They are known as **employability skills**. The employability skills required for the hair and beauty sectors are:

- Good communication skills.
- A willingness to learn.
- Self-manager.
- Teamworker.
- Good client care skills.
- A positive attitude.
- Good personal ethics.
- Creative.
- Prepared to work flexible working hours.
- Leadership qualities.

Career progression in hair and beauty

Qualification level	Training programme	Job role
Honours degree in management.	• University	Industry consultant Inspector Education manager
Foundation degree in hair and beauty management.	• Work based – working in a salon • College programme • University programme	Salon or spa owner**** Salon or spa manager**** Teacher* Lecturer* Advanced practitioner***
Level 3 programmes in hair and beauty. This is the expected standard for anyone who wishes to work in a salon or spa.	• Apprenticeship • College-based programmes	Senior**: *Hairdresser* *Barber* *Therapist* *Nail technician* *Receptionist* Trainer* Assessor* Sales representative Manufacturer technician
Level 2 programmes in hair and beauty. This is a basic qualification for junior level staff.	• Apprenticeship • College-based programmes	Junior: *Hairdresser* *Barber* *Therapist* *Nail technician* *Receptionist*
Young apprenticeship in hair and beauty.	• School- and college-based programme with 50 days' work experience	Salon assistant in hair and beauty
Foundation programmes in hair and beauty.	• School- and college-based programmes with some work experience	Work experience

* Job roles like this will require additional training and you will have to complete more qualifications, such as teacher training or assessor qualifications.

** If you are a senior stylist you can work in lots of different types of salon. They can be on the high street, in department stores, on board cruise liners, in hospitals and care homes. Hair and beauty qualifications from the UK are recognized in many counties, so you could work in locations around the world. You could also work as a freelance hairdresser, beauty therapist or nail technician. Some very talented people may find work as a film or TV hairdresser or make-up artist.

*** Advanced practitioners work in some very highly skilled areas of beauty therapy, for example, in laser hair removal or semi-permanent make-up. For these jobs you would need to complete some additional and very specialized training.

**** If you are a salon or spa owner or manager you will benefit from studying for additional, management qualifications. Higher education qualification such as foundation degrees can be studied part time at a college or university while you work in the salon.

Do you think you have the employability skills to work in the hair and beauty sector? Is a job in hair and beauty for you? Complete this quiz and find out.

Circle A or B which is *more* like you in each section.

Communication

1	I only like to talk to people I know	A
	I like to talk to anyone	B
2	People think I talk a great deal	A
	People like talking to me	B
3	I am only happy when I am talking to others	A
	I like to listen to other people	B

Willingness to learn

1	I am curious and like to learn about new things	A
	I am only interested in the things I already know about	B
2	I try hard with things that take a long time to learn	A
	I get bored if I can't learn something quickly	B
3	I am not happy unless something is perfect	A
	I cut corners if something takes too long to complete	B

Self-manager

1	I am very organized and would know exactly where to find a particular item of clothing or textbook	A
	I am not very organized and would have to search to find an item clothing or textbook	B
2	I am up to date with all my school or college work	A
	I have several pieces of work to hand in	B

| 3 | My friends often ask me to help them with their problems | A |
| | I often ask my friends to help me with my problems | B |

Teamwork

1	I like to be in control of a group of people	A
	I work well on my own and with a group of people	B
2	I don't like to listen to those who criticize me	A
	If one of my friends disagrees with something I am doing, I like to hear their views	B
3	I don't like it if others do better than me	A
	When I work with others, I enjoy seeing them do well	B

Client care

1	If someone pushes in front of me in a queue, I would think of a reason why they had done this	A
	If someone pushes in front of me in a queue I would immediately ask them to go to the back	B
2	I like to gain feedback from others about work I have done	A
	I am not interested in what others think about my work	B
3	When I am in a situation where there is an argument, I do all I can to calm the situation	A
	I enjoy getting in situations that cause arguments because it is interesting	B

Positive attitude

| 1 | If something does not work the first time, I am happy to try again | A |
| | I get very frustrated if I can't get something to work | B |

2	I recognize that some criticism of my work will help me to improve	A
	I get upset when I have worked hard and someone does not like what I have done	B
3	I am aware that others may have a different point of view from me, and can still be right	A
	If people do not agree with me, then they are wrong	B

Personal ethics

1	I would hope that no one would notice if I was late for school or college	A
	If I know I am going to be late for school or college, I would always let someone know	B
2	I only like being with people who enjoy the same things as me	A
	I enjoy being with people who are different from me	B
3	If I found something very valuable in the street, I would keep it if no one noticed that I had picked it up	A
	If I found something very valuable in the street, I would hand it in at the police station	B

Creativity

1	If I have a new project, to complete I like to imagine how the end result will look	A
	I dislike experimenting with different ideas and don't like starting new projects	B
2	I enjoy trying new things	A
	I prefer to continue with work that I know and understand	B
3	I love to show others my new ideas	A
	If I have a new idea, I like to keep it to myself	B

Flexible working

1	I like to complete one job before I begin another	A
	I am able to work on more than one project at a time	B
2	I prefer routine	A
	I don't mind if my routine is changed	B
3	I prefer work that is routine	A
	I prefer work that is challenging	B

Leadership

1	When working in a group I am happy to give others tasks to do	A
	I prefer others to tell me what to do	B
2	When planning work I can see where one task can link with another	A
	I like to plan one job at a time	B
3	I enjoy helping others to achieve	A
	I find having to help others frustrating	B

Results for the employability skills test

When you have completed all the questions, find out if you have the employability skills required to work in the hair and beauty sectors.

Communication Having good communication skills is probably the most important of all the employability skills.

Mainly As   *You need to improve your communication skills if you want to work in the hair and beauty sector. Being able to communicate includes listening as well as talking to a range of different people.*

Mainly Bs   *You have communication skills that would be useful for the hair and beauty sector.*

Willingness to learn The skills, theory and knowledge you will study if you work in the hair and beauty sectors are not easy to learn. So you have to be *willing to learn.*

Mainly As *You show the willingness to learn what is required for the hair and beauty sector.*

Mainly Bs *The skills and knowledge required to work in the hair and beauty sector take many years to gain – and then you have to keep learning for the rest of your working life. If you are the type of person who is only satisfied when you can do a job quickly, then perhaps the hair and beauty sectors are not for you.*

Self-manager You have to be good at planning your own time if you want to work in the hair and beauty sectors.

Mainly As *You show signs that you are capable of being a self-manager.*

Mainly Bs *You need to be able to manage your time and learning if you are going to succeed in the hair and beauty sector.*

Teamwork If you go to a busy salon there will be a team of people to look after you. Each person is working with others to ensure that you have a pleasant experience. Teamwork is also about having respect, consideration and understanding for others.

Mainly As *Teamwork involves being adaptable and listening to the views of others. Perhaps you would be more suited to a career where you can sometimes work on your own.*

Mainly Bs *You have the capability to successfully work in a team with other people, which is a skill required for the hair and beauty sectors.*

Client care Client care is very important and can be anything from providing a full treatment or service or offering to make a drink for a client.

Mainly As *You have social awareness, and you are sensitive to social situations, which is a useful skill for client care.*

Mainly Bs *Having a lack of tolerance is not good when developing customer care skills, so perhaps the hair and beauty sectors are not for you.*

Positive attitude Because the training you need for the hair and beauty sectors is long and sometimes difficult, you need to show that you are patient, tolerant and have a good sense of humour.

Mainly As *You show that you have drive and commitment as well as tolerance, which are all useful qualities for the hair and beauty sectors.*

Mainly Bs *You need to improve your skills of patience and tolerance if you want to succeed in the hair and beauty sectors.*

IT'S A FACT!

Client care is one employability skill that is linked to many of the others. For example, you cannot achieve good client care if you have poor communication skills or there are members of the salon team who do not work well together.

Personal ethics When you work in the hair and beauty sectors, clients will trust you. You must never tell others about the personal conversations you have with your clients. Personal ethics is also about being honest and reliable.

> **Mainly As**   *You need to improve your honesty and reliability if you want to work in the hair and beauty sectors.*
>
> **Mainly Bs**   *You show signs that you have a good work ethic and social and cultural awareness, which are required in the hair and beauty sectors.*

Creativity Being creative is a major advantage if you want to work in the hair and beauty sectors. You need to be brave and experiment with different ideas.

> **Mainly As**   *You have signs of creativity and the ability to inspire others, which is a good skill to have if you want to work in the hair and beauty sectors.*
>
> **Mainly Bs**   *To be successful in the hair and beauty sectors you must be able to share your original ideas.*

Flexible working Those who work in the hair and beauty sectors do not have 9–5 jobs. Your work cannot end until your client is finished. You may not be able to have weekends off and you may be expected to work in shifts, which can include working in the evenings.

> **Mainly As**   *Your rigid nature will restrict you if you work in the hair and beauty sectors.*
>
> **Mainly Bs**   *You shows signs that you have a flexible approach to work, which is an attribute that is required for the hair and beauty sectors.*

Leadership If you can lead others you could have a very successful career in the hair and beauty sectors. And the good thing is that you do not have wait until you are a manager to do this. Some leadership is required right at the very beginning of your training.

SIGNPOST
PLTS

Independent enquirer
Reflective learner

> **Mainly As**   *You have qualities that can be developed into true leadership skills, which are required when working in the hair and beauty sectors.*
>
> **Mainly Bs**   *You need to develop you leadership skills if you want to work in the hair and beauty sectors.*

SIGNPOST
FUNCTIONAL
SKILL

English
When you read the information for the employability skills quiz you will be able to:
E3   read and understand the purpose and content of straightforward texts to understand the main points
L1   read and understand the purpose and content of straightforward texts to understand the text in detail.

Where you can find more information about careers in the hair and beauty sector

To find out more about careers in hair and beauty you can talk to your careers teachers at school or college. They will be able to tell you more about the different types of training programme you can do.

You can make a visit to your local career office and talk to a personal advisor.

WEB LINK

Look at the Connexions website for all sorts of useful career advice: **http://www.connexions-direct.com/**. You can try out the quizzes to see which job would be best for you.

What you have learnt

Job roles in the hair and beauty sector

- There are six industries in the hair and beauty sector. They are:
  ○ Hairdressing.
  ○ Barbering.
  ○ African-Caribbean hairdressing and barbering.
  ○ Beauty therapy.
  ○ Nail services.
  ○ Spa therapy.
- The six different industries have different types of salon.

WEB LINK

Look at this web link to see the career progression paths for all the hair and beauty sectors. You can print off the career leaflets for all the hair and beauty sectors and keep them in your file. You will also find the answers to frequently asked questions. Go to **http://www.habia.org/** and then click on 'Careers'.

Working patterns in the hair and beauty sector

- Working in hair and beauty is not a 9–5 job.
- You may have to work at the weekends and in the evenings.

Career opportunities and progression in hair and beauty

- It takes a long time to train for jobs in the hair and beauty sector.
- There are many different career opportunities, such as:
  ○ Junior stylist, therapist or nail technician.
  ○ Senior stylist, therapist or nail technician.
  ○ Assessor, teacher, trainer, lecturer.
  ○ Salon or spa owner or manager.
  ○ Advanced practitioner.
  ○ Industry consultant.
  ○ Education manager.
  ○ Inspector.

WEB LINK

This web link will lead you to a Habia Student Handbook for hairdressers and beauty therapists. It is full of useful career progression information: **http://www.habia.org/uploads/student_handbook.pdf**

WEB LINK

For more information about work experience in the hair and beauty sectors, read this Learner Handbook: **http://www.habia.org/uploads/8106_Learner_HB_A4.pdf**

- You need to have good employability skills when working in the hair and beauty sectors. The skills you need are:

  - Good communication skills.

  - A willingness to learn.

  - Self-manager.

  - Teamworker.

  - Good client care skills.

  - A positive attitude.

  - Good personal ethics.

  - Creative.

  - Prepared to work flexible working hours.

  - Leadership qualities.

Pay structure in the hair and beauty sector

- When you first start your training the pay may be low.

- You will earn more as you gain more skills and progress to higher level jobs.

- You will earn more through commission.

Learning programmes in hair and beauty

You can follow a hair and beauty programme in a school, college or as an apprentice.

Employment rights and responsibilities in the hair and beauty sector

As an apprentice you will learn about your employment rights and responsibilities.

Where you can find more information about careers

- You can find out more about careers in the hair and beauty sectors by:

  - Talking to your careers teacher.

  - Speaking to a personal advisor at Connexions.

  - Visiting the Connexions website.

  - Visiting the Habia website.

ASSESSMENT ACTIVITIES

Activity 1 E3 – L1

These are multiple choice questions. Read through each question carefully. When you have finished, tick the correct answer.

1 In the hair and beauty sector there are:

    a. Six industries.   c. Four industries.

    b. Seven industries.   d. Three industries.

2 If you are carrying out a facial hair trim, you are:

    a. A nail technician.   c. A barber.

    b. A beauty therapist.   d. A hairdresser.

3 Thermal styling is most likely to be carried out in:

    a. A beauty therapy salon.

    b. A salon that specializes in African type hair.

    c. A barber's shop.

    d. A day spa in a country hotel.

4 If you are freelance barber you will:

    a. Cut the hair of women and girls.

    b. Work in a barber's shop.

    c. Cut African type hair.

    d. Travel around to visit your clients.

5 The music played in a beauty therapy salon is likely to be:

    a. Loud.   c. Modern.

    b. Relaxing.   d. Traditional.

6 Work-based learning is the term given to:

    a. College courses.

    b. School programmes.

    c. Apprenticeships.

    d. Hairdressing.

7 ERR stands for:

    a. Employment responsibilities and regulations.

    b. Employment rules and rights.

    c. Employment regulations and rules.

    d. Employment rights and responsibilities.

8 All those working in a hair or beauty salon as senior stylists, therapists or technicians should be qualified at:

    a. Level 3.   c. Level 1.

    b. Level 4.   d. Level 2.

9 Willingness to learn, client care and teamwork are all examples of:

    a. Certificates.

    b. Learning programmes.

    c. Employability skills.

    d. Qualifications.

10 Training to work in the hair and beauty sectors:

    a. Takes a long time and you never stop learning.

    b. Is quick and very easy.

    c. Can be completed in under 6 months.

    d. Takes one year to complete the qualification.

Activity 2 E1–L1

Match the treatment or service with the job role

Draw an arrow to the person who is most likely to carry out the treatment or service.

Cutting hair in 3D designs	Nail technician
Relaxing hair	Barber
Indian head massage	Hairdresser
Waxing	Spa therapist
Dressing long hair	Beauty therapist
Extending nails	African type hairdresser

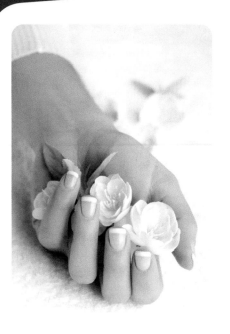

2

Personal and social development

" A person who has never made a mistake never tried anything new.

ALBERT EINSTEIN

In this chapter you are going to learn about:

● The importance of teamwork in the hair and beauty sector.

● Presenting a professional image.

● Personal hygiene.

● The expected behaviour required when working in a salon.

● Using communication in the hair and beauty sector.

● Working on reception.

● Managing your money.

Introduction

First impressions count. Remember that the way you look and behave will form a lasting impression and enable people to make a judgement about you.

The way you speak and act with others is very important when working in the hair and beauty industry. In a salon you will need to build relationships with both your team members and the clients who visit. You will also learn about the importance of teamwork and why it is important to work with and support your team members when working in the salon.

In this chapter you will also learn how to help develop your own skills such as building relationships when working with other people, and how preparing yourself and presenting a good professional image can help to give you confidence.

You will need to understand the different methods of communicating and how you can use communication skills to give a good impression of yourself so that people have confidence in you.

When you read this chapter you will learn about the different skills you need to successfully work on a salon reception, from greeting clients to taking payments, and the different types of technology that can be used. It will also give you ideas that you can use in your general life, such as how to manage your money.

The importance of teamwork in the hair and beauty sector

There are lots of different jobs that need to be done in a salon; each person working in a salon must have the skills and knowledge to carry out some of those jobs.

In the salon it is important that everyone helps and supports each other, this is called **teamwork**.

Good teamwork is very important when working in a salon. Everyone has to work together to make sure the client enjoys their visit and will be happy to come back. Teamwork ensures that the salon runs smoothly, it gives clients a positive impression of the salon and the people who work in it.

So it doesn't matter what level you are or what job you do in a salon, everyone needs to work together to be successful.

Job roles found in a hair and beauty salon include:

- *A salon junior or a young apprentice.* In this role you are just starting your career. You will be learning new things all the time and helping senior members of the team to do their jobs. This will include:
  - Getting the work area ready for the next client.
  - Hanging up clients' coats and looking after them while they are waiting in the reception area.
  - Making drinks.
  - Supporting the stylist or therapist if needed while they are working with a **client**.
  - Helping at reception.
- *A junior stylist or therapist.* In this role you will have just completed all your basic training to become a therapist or stylist. You will be starting to build up your own clientele.

  Job roles for a junior stylist will include:
  - Shampooing and conditioning hair.
  - Cutting and styling hair.
  - Colouring hair.
  - Perming or straightening hair.
  - Dressing hair.

WHAT'S NEXT?

When you progress to Level 2 you will learn more about all the different technical skills that you will need to become a successful stylist or therapist.

Job roles for a junior therapist will include:

○ Carrying out facials.

○ Applying make-up for different occasions.

○ Removing unwanted hair by waxing or plucking.

○ Carrying out manicures and pedicures.

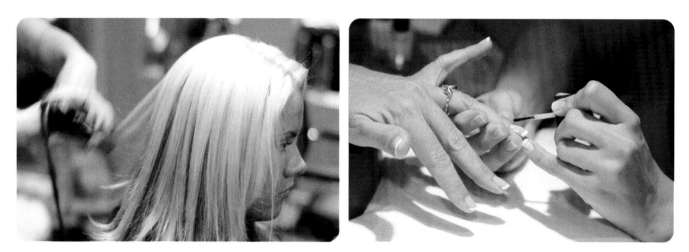

A stylist and beauty therapist working

● *A senior stylist or therapist.* In this role you will be very busy with clients carrying out all the different services or treatments. Some of these **treatments** and **services** will be difficult to carry out. You will need help from your other team members to make sure everything runs smoothly for your clients.

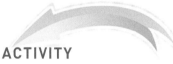

ACTIVITY

Work in a team to identify and discuss some of the different services and treatments that would be carried out by a senior stylist or therapist. You can then use the table below to write down your findings.

Services carried out by a senior stylist	Treatments carried out by a senior therapist

SIGNPOST
PLTS

Teamworker
Effective participators

English

SIGNPOST
FUNCTIONAL
SKILL

When you use the table to write down your findings, you will able to show you can:

E3   plan, draft and organize writing; sequence writing logically and clearly

L1   present information in a logical sequence.

- *A receptionist*. In this role you will be very busy making sure that the clients are looked after.

  Job roles for a receptionist include:

  ○ Making appointments for clients.

  ○ Greeting clients and looking after them at reception.

  ○ Taking client payments.

  ○ Taking and passing on messages.

  ○ Dealing with different types of visit.

  ○ Displaying and maintaining retail stock.

- *A salon manager*. In this role you will be very busy making sure that the salon runs smoothly and is making enough money to employ the staff it needs to be successful.

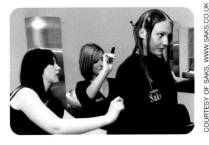

An apprentice hairdresser

First impressions are important and they do count. Clients will make a judgement about what they see and hear in the first few minutes of entering the salon. They will notice and take account of the way they are greeted and looked after as they arrive, they will notice how the salon looks. Is it clean and tidy? They will also see how the team in the salon work together, talk and relate to each other, and how well the services or treatments are carried out.

Everyone working in the salon must make a **positive impression**. The way you present yourself and act will form part of the clients' overall judgement of the salon.

IT'S A FACT!

Clients come to a salon for a number of reasons:

- To improve their appearance.

- To improve their **well-being**.

- To relax and enjoy the experience.

Presenting a professional image

The way you look, the clothes you wear and the actions you take will all send messages to the outside world about how you want people to see you. To make an overall good impression it is not only important to dress correctly for the occasion; it is also about thinking from 'top to toe' and making sure your overall appearance is good:

- Your clothes and shoes need to be well looked after, clean and in good repair.

- Your hair needs to be clean and styled.

- Your skin should look fresh and clean.

- Any make-up should be well applied.

ACTIVITY

Within a team discuss the good and bad points about wearing a uniform.

SIGNPOST FUNCTIONAL SKILLS

SIGNPOST PLTS

Teamworker
Effective participators

● Your hands and nails should be well maintained.

● Nail polish, if worn, should not be worn or chipped.

Most hair and beauty salons will have a type of uniform. Beauty therapists usually wear a formal uniform to portray an image of harmony and uniformity. In hairdressing stylists do not usually have a **formal** uniform.

English
When you discuss the good and bad points about wearing a uniform you will:
E3 respond appropriately to others and make some extended contributions in familiar formal or informal discussions and exchanges
L1 take full part in formal or informal discussions and exchanges that include unfamiliar subjects.

Some salons will have a set colour theme, where the staff all wear the same colour, in other salons you may be given total freedom to wear what you want.

No matter what you are wearing, your appearance will send messages to the client. A clean and well-presented outfit will give the client confidence. If clothes are dirty and soiled, not only does it give clients a bad impression, but it can also be embarrassing and upsetting to clients and your team members if that means you also smell sweaty.

A stylist looking dishevelled and a stylist looking well presented A therapist looking well presented and a therapist looking dishevelled.

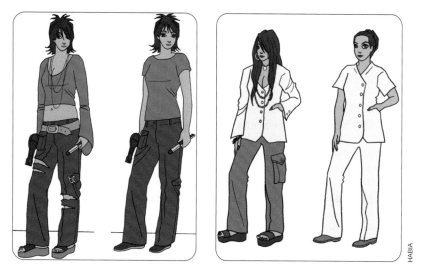

Personal hygiene

It is important that you maintain high standards of personal **hygiene**. Body hygiene is achieved through daily washing to remove stale sweat, dirt and any bacteria, all of which create **body odour (BO)**:

● Underwear should be clean and fresh each day.

● Teeth should be cleaned regularly, especially after eating.

- Use breath fresheners or mouthwash to help freshen your breath.

- Antiperspirants or deodorants should be used under the arms to help reduce perspiration and the smell of sweat.

Hands should be washed regularly throughout the day, especially after visiting the toilet, before eating food or carrying out a service or treatment.

How to wash hands

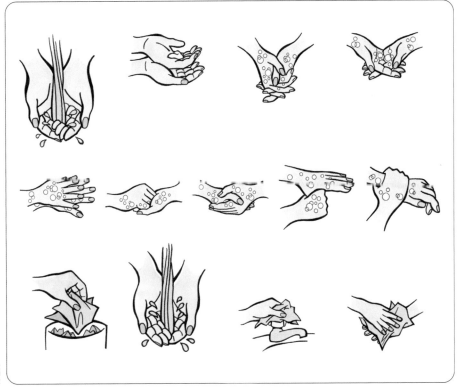

HABIA

When working in the hair and beauty sector you are working with people all day and you need to make sure that you treat all clients in the same professional way. Remember that you need to look and act professionally.

Think about the following when meeting a client:

- Greet them with a smile – think of clients as being someone you know or your friend. This will help you to relax and you will naturally start to smile.

- Don't cross your arms, it can look defensive.

- Make eye contact when talking or listening to a client.

- Stand up straight and don't slouch.

- Be positive and helpful.

Behaviour expectations for the hair and beauty sector

Positive messages are also given by the way that you behave.

The way you present yourself and behave at work will show your professionalism. To be a good employee and team member it is important that you get on well with the people you work with. You have to be positive and focused on the job, enjoy what you are doing and be supportive, open and helpful to other team members.

Most salons will have rules that are written down in **work policies** that cover different situations, such as health and safety or **personal conduct**.

A policy on personal conduct may include:

- Time schedules for working.
- Reporting in when you are sick and cannot come to work.
- Dress code.
- How to behave.
- Salon's rule on smoking.
- Where and when eating and drinking can take place.

SIGNPOST ERR

As part of employment rights and responsibilities when working in a salon you will need to have a basic knowledge on issues relating to your employment terms and conditions and disciplinary procedures. This will include:

- What is included in a contract of employment.
- Holiday entitlements.
- Company pension scheme arrangements.
- The salon's rules and regulations/codes of practice/work policies.
- Procedures to take if you have a problem at work or cannot come to work.
- Your employer's expectations in terms of behaviour, conduct and performance.
- The steps taken as part of a disciplinary process.
- Who to approach if you are worried about anything to do with work or your training.

Using communication in the hair and beauty sector

Communication is the passing on of information, ideas or feelings. How and when you do this will affect your relationships with other people.

There are different methods of communicating and it is important that you use all of them to make sure that people understand what you are saying or doing.

When carrying out a client consultation you communicate to first make the client feel relaxed, and second to find out exactly what your client wants or expects from you.

Verbal communication

Verbal communication is about speaking and using your voice to get information across. One-to-one communication is very important in the hair and beauty sector. Your voice can express your attitude and your emotions.

To communicate effectively you should:

- Keep information simple.
- Speak clearly.
- Vary your voice tone, pitch and volume.
- Speak courteously and with confidence.
- Do not use slang.
- Never speak while you are eating or chewing.

Non-verbal communication

There are a lot of different ways in which we communicate non-verbally. These may include such things as:

- Making gestures and facial expressions.
- Using eye contact.
- Clothes and accessories.
- Writing down information.

When you are communicating with your clients, your message is delivered in three ways:

- Your body language.
- Your tone of voice.
- The words you use.

Body language is a very important part of communication. The way you stand, make eye contact and use your facial expressions will send a message to people around you. Think about how you look when you are happy. You smile and your whole face lights up. When you are sad your mouth is down-turned and your eyes appear dull.

Being able to interpret different signals and understand how to act on them will make it a lot easier to work with clients. You will be able to reassure or relax a client who is feeling worried and this all helps to build a good relationship.

IT'S A FACT!

Personal space is the invisible boundary that surrounds a person's body. That space ensures the person feels and remains comfortable when in the company of other people, particularly if they are strangers.

SIGNPOST PLTS

Teamworker

Effective participators

SIGNPOST FUNCTIONAL SKILLS

ACTIVITY

In a group discuss how you act and communicate differently with different people. This could include:

● Your parents.

● Your friends.

● Strangers.

Non-verbal communication also includes listening skills. You need good listening skills so that you can find out what the client wants. You also need reading skills so that you can read manufacturer's instructions and client record cards to find out about important information so that you work safely.

English
When taking part in a discussion, you will:
E3 respond appropriately to others and make some extended contributions in familiar formal and informal discussions and exchanges
L1 take full part in formal and informal discussions and exchanges that include unfamiliar subjects.

Physical communication

Physical communication is about touching people and being in someone's personal space. In the hair and beauty sector you will always use physical communication because you will have to touch people.

When you first start your career in hair or beauty, touching people can be quite frightening or threatening. It is important to learn how to enter a person's space without their feeling uncomfortable. Lightly putting your hand on a client's arm or shoulder when you are talking to them or during a **consultation** will help make the client feel more relaxed.

Asking questions

You will need to ask lots of questions and listen to your client's answers during the consultation. It is important to use a variety of different questions so that you gather lots of correct information. The use of open and closed questions will help you do this.

Open questions

Open questions can start with any of the following words:

● Who

● What

● Where

● Would

● When

● How.

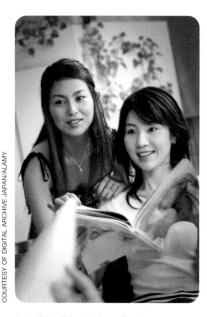

A stylist talking to her client

Questions starting with these words will encourage your client to give you more information than a 'yes' and a 'no' response.

Types of open questions you can ask your client:

- What would you like done today?
- Can you tell me what you do not like about your hair?
- What is your skincare routine at home?
- When did you last visit the salon?
- Can you tell me a little bit about your lifestyle?

Closed questions

Closed questions are used when you want to gain a limited response such as 'yes' or 'no'. You would use this type of questioning to confirm your understanding of your client's requirements. Types of closed questions you could ask your client:

- Are you having your hair cut today?
- Do you want your nails filed any shorter?
- Do you want to look at a style book?
- Is the water too hot?

English
When you are taking part in a discussion on different methods of communication, you will:
E3   respond appropriately to others and make some extended contributions in familiar formal or informal discussions and exchanges
L1   take full part in formal or informal discussions and exchanges that include unfamiliar subjects.

ACTIVITY

With a partner, practise different methods of communication. Pick a topic from the list below that you would like to discuss. Can you identify the different types of communication skill that are being used?

- Favourite type of food.
- Favourite type of music.
- Favourite film.

SIGNPOST PLTS

Teamworker
Effective participators

SIGNPOST FUNCTIONAL SKILLS

Working on reception

The reception area is a very busy place, with clients coming and going, telephones ringing, clients wanting to make appointments and paying their bills. The reception area will have an area for clients to wait for their appointments, where they can read magazines and have a drink. It needs to look clean and comfortable at all times. It is the receptionist's job to ensure that the reception area runs smoothly and efficiently all day. They have to be good organizers as they need to manage time and work schedules for themselves and the stylists or therapists.

TOP TIP

During the consultation, a hairdresser will sit next to their clients so that the client feels at ease, rather than standing over them.

ACTIVITY

Create a hairstyle or beauty treatment file that could be kept in the reception area for clients to look at while they are waiting for their appointment.

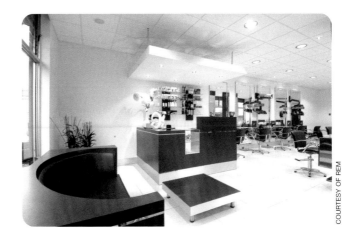

A reception area

SIGNPOST PLTS

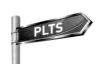

Creative thinker
Reflective learner
Self-manager

Receptionists need to be confident, friendly and good communicators. They are the first point of contact for a client, either face-to-face or on the telephone.

Communication skills are very important for receptionists. This will include verbal and non-verbal communication as well as written communication. Many receptionists also have to use information communication technology (ICT) as part of their daily work. They may have to use a computer to look after client information that is stored on a database or schedule **appointments.**

The salon manager can also use information from the computer to find out how well the salon is doing.

Computerized appointment system from shortcuts

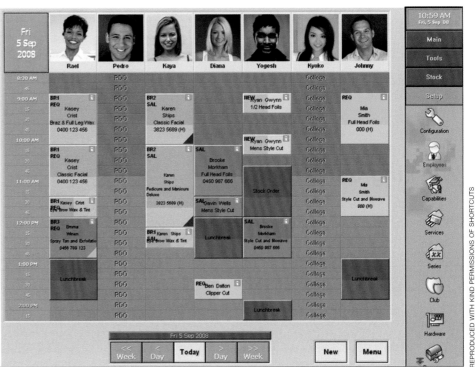

Answering the telephone

A receptionist will answer most telephone calls received in a salon. However, not all salons have a receptionist, so it is important that everyone in the salon is trained to use and answer the telephone.

Using the right tone of voice to answer the telephone is very important, your voice should sound welcoming and friendly. When speaking, make sure you speak clearly and do not mumble or speak too quickly. You need to alter the tone of your voice so that you sound interested in the caller.

Taking messages

At reception you will often take, record and pass on messages. It is important that you take the details of the message clearly and **accurately** in order to maintain effective communication within the salon. It is also important that you only give the information to the person it is meant for.

Messages must be clearly written and include, as a minimum, the following information:

- Who the message is for.
- Who has taken the message.
- The date and time the message was taken.
- What the message is.
- Any action required.
- If the message is urgent.
- How to reply to the message (contact details).

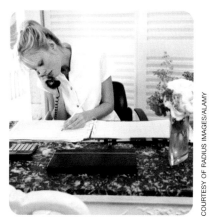

Receptionist answering the telephone

IT'S A FACT!

Smiling when answering the telephone will help you have a friendly tone of voice.

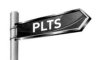

Telephone and message pad

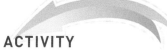

ACTIVITY

Within a team, practise answering the telephone. Take it in turns to take a message and to write down the information that needs to be passed on someone. Make sure you cover all the minimum information required to ensure that you have given clear and accurate information.

SIGNPOST PLTS

Teamwork
Effective participators

SIGNPOST FUNCTIONAL SKILLS

English

When you practise answering the telephone and write down messages, you will:

E3 respond appropriately to others and make some extended contributions in familiar formal or informal discussions and exchanges

L1 take full part in formal or informal discussions and exchanges that include unfamiliar subjects

E3 write texts with some adaption to the intended audience

L1 write a range of texts to communicate information, ideas and opinions, using formats and styles suitable for the purpose and audience.

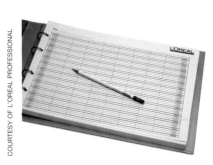

Paper-based appointment book

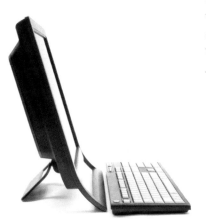

Computer-based appointment system

Making appointments

The appointment system is important to any salon. It is essential that appointments are made clearly and accurately. If there are mistakes made when making an appointment this will affect the smooth running of the salon. Clients may have to wait for their service or treatment to be carried out or they may leave because they cannot wait.

Each salon will have different services and treatments on offer and they will have different **abbreviations** that are used when making appointments. Different stylists or therapists will have different skills and skill levels. You will have to get to know how your salon appointment system works so that you can successfully book appointments.

Making an appointment does not have to be difficult. You have to learn about the services carried out in the salon, the timings required to carry out those services and the abbreviations used in the appointment system. You must do it carefully and accurately as the information will tell the stylist or therapist who their client is and what service or treatment to prepare for.

To make an appointment you will need to have the following information:

- Date and time the client would like the appointment.
- Service or treatment they are booking for.
- Name of the preferred stylist or therapist.
- The name of the client.
- The client's contact details.

ACTIVITY

Working on your own, identify the abbreviations used for the range of services and treatments offered in the salon. These abbreviations will then be used when making appointments. Some examples are:

Service	Abbreviation
Cut and blow dry	CB/D
Highlights	H/L
Manicure	Man

Once you have identified the abbreviations present them in a simple table format.

SIGNPOST PLTS

Independent enquirer

SIGNPOST FUNCTIONAL SKILLS

ICT

When you are presenting information in a table format you will interact with ICT systems to meet given needs at E3 and Level 1.

ACTIVITY

Find out about the different treatments or services that are offered in a hair or beauty salon. Find out how long each treatment or service takes and how much they cost. When booking the treatment or service remember to find out if there is an additional time gap required for a second part to the service. For example, if carrying out a colour service will the client need a second appointment for a cut and blow dry?

Fill in the chart with the information you have found:

Treatment or service	Time required	Gap required in the appointment system if there are two parts to the service	Cost

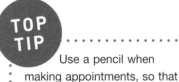

WHAT'S NEXT?

When you progress to Level 2 reception duties you will learn about how to deal with clients in the reception area and how to successfully make client appointments and take payments.

TOP TIP

Use a pencil when making appointments, so that you can rub out cancellations or make changes.

SIGNPOST PLTS

PLTS

Independent enquirer
Self-manager

English
When completing the chart on different treatments and services, you will:

E3 plan, draft and organize writing; sequence writing logically and clearly

L1 write clearly and coherently, including an appropriate level of detail; present information in a logical sequence.

SIGNPOST FUNCTIONAL SKILLS

Taking payments

When a service or treatment is complete it will be time for the client to pay the bill. You will need to calculate how much the client needs to pay. Make sure that you double-check your calculation before telling the client how much to pay.

Clients may wish to pay their bill by cash, by **debit** or **credit card**, by cheque or they may have been given a gift voucher as a present.

WHAT'S NEXT?

When you progress to Level 2 reception duties you will learn about how to take payments using all the different methods.

IT'S A FACT!

Being able to use maths in a salon is very important. Not only do you need to be able to work out client bills and take payments but you also will need to work out percentages when mixing products together or measuring out the amount of products to use.

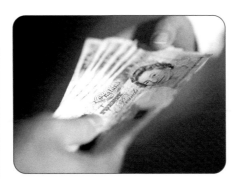

Cash payment

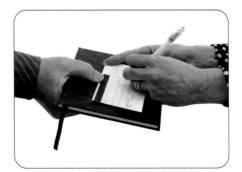

Cheque payment

ACTIVITY

With a partner, take it in turns to be the client and the receptionist. Then take it in turns to practise calculating a client's bill and taking cash payment. Don't forget to use your communication skills.

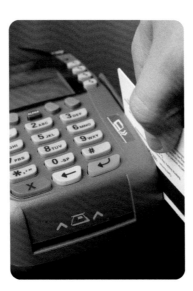

Credit card payment

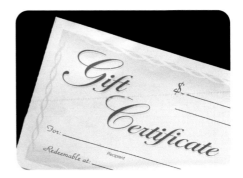

Gift voucher

SIGNPOST PLTS

Teamwork
Effective participators

SIGNPOST FUNCTIONAL SKILLS

English

When carrying out reception duties, you will:

E3 respond appropriately to others and make some extended contributions in familiar formal or informal discussions and exchanges

L1 take full part in formal or informal discussions and exchanges that include unfamiliar subjects.

SIGNPOST FUNCTIONAL SKILLS

Maths

When you are preparing and calculating a client's bill you will be representing and analysing mathematics to obtain simple calculations involving money at E3 and L1.

Shortcuts report for employee takings

Employee Services Breakdown

Current Month: 01/02/2008 to 20/02/2008

All prices are inc GST

	Clients	Ladies	Mens	Kids	H/Lights	Semis	Tints	Perms	Treat	Exten	Models
Today	6	5	1	0	0	0	0	0	0	0	0
Business	23	15	4	3	5	0	5	0	0	0	0
Week	26	19	3	2	0	0	0	0	0	0	0
Business	90	61	15	5	17	1	19	0	0	2	0
Month	81	65	7	3	1	0	2	0	0	0	0
Business	369	263	49	20	84	9	81	0	0	6	0

Employee Pounds Breakdown

	Service #	Rebook #	Retail #	Service £	Retail £	Sundry £	Total £	Avg/Client £	Points #
Today	6 (6)	0	3	£139.73	£38.85	£0.00	£178.58	£29.76	0
Business	33	0	6	£992.58	£67.70	£0.00	£1,060.28	£46.10	0
Week	26 (27)	0	6	£721.93	£80.70	£0.00	£802.63	£30.87	0
Business	122	0	23	£3,765.36	£382.90	£0.00	£4,148.26	£46.09	0
Month	82 (84)	1	9	£2,358.19	£121.55	£0.00	£2,479.74	£30.61	0
Business	493	1	73	£15,045.16	£1,247.26	£0.00	£16,292.42	£44.15	0

IT'S A FACT!

Many stylists and therapists receive commission as part of their salary. Commission is based on the amount of money their clients spend in the salon. This is why it is important to accurately calculate client bills and record the information for individual members of the team.

Managing your money

Money is important to us all, without it you cannot live. Where would you live? How would you eat and what would you wear? We all work to make money. It is up to you how you spend your money. You have to make sure that you plan how to spend it and if you have any money to save. This is called a budget plan.

A **budget plan** will help you organize your money. It will help you work out how much money you have left after you have paid for your living expenses.

Everyone will have a different budget plan depending on what their individual priorities are. Some people will need to budget for a car, others for a house mortgage. Some people may only be able to afford to get their hair cut every three months, while other people will budget to have it cut every six weeks.

ACTIVITY

Using the budget plan and information below can you work out how much money you will have left to spend on yourself after paying your living expenses?

You take home £400.00 per month for your salary. With that money you need to pay your living expenses before you can spend any remaining money.

1 How much money do you spend on living expenses each month?

2 How much money do you have left?

3 If you saved £50.00 per month from your remaining money, how much money would you have left?

4 If, instead of saving your money, you decide to buy and run a car that will cost you £120.00 per month, how much money would you then have left?

5 If you bought a car this would save money on your budgeted travel costs. How much money would you save per month?

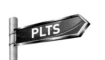

6 If you did not buy a car how would you spend your remaining monthly savings among
the remaining three headings of Savings, Loans and Other expenses?

Monthly living expenses	Outgoing costs
Rent including services	£150.00
Food	£45.00
Travel	£ 25.00
Entertainment	£16.00
Clothes	£20.00
Savings	nil
Loans	nil
Other expenses	nil

Maths

When you are calculating a budget plan you will be representing and analysing
mathematics to obtain simple calculations involving money at E3 and L1.

Usually, when you get paid for your work in a salon this is done on a set
date in the month and the money will go into your bank account. The salon
owner will need to have your banking details so that they can make sure the
money goes directly into your bank. You will receive a pay slip from your employer that will explain how much money you have earned and if there have
been any reductions taken off for income tax and national insurance. It will
also show you money that has been removed if you have been sick and unable to work.

Some employers may pay you on a weekly basis in cash, you will still receive a
pay slip and you may want to have a bank account to put your money in to keep
it safe and help you save.

ICT

When you are looking at websites for information from different banks you will interact
with ICT for a given purpose and you will be able to recognize and use interface
features. **E3** and **L1**

Useful websites for finding out about starting a bank account:

www.natwest.co.uk
www.hsbc.co.uk
www.barclays.co.uk
www.halifax.co.uk
www.rbs.co.uk

What you have learnt

- The importance of teamwork in the hair and beauty sector:

  ○ The different types of job role.

  ○ The importance of teamwork.

- Presenting a professional image:

  ○ What you wear and how this reflects the image of the salon.

  ○ Personal hygiene.

  ○ Behaviour expectations for the hair and beauty sector.

- Using communication in the hair and beauty sector:

  ○ Understanding and using verbal and non-verbal communication.

  ○ What is meant by physical communication.

  ○ How to use open and closed questions.

- How to work on reception:

  ○ The role of reception.

  ○ The role of the receptionist.

  ○ How to answering the telephone.

  ○ How to take a message.

  ○ The importance of making appointments correctly.

  ○ The importance of taking payments.

- How to manage your money:

  ○ What is a budget plan and how to use one.

  ○ How and when you get paid.

ASSESSMENT ACTIVITIES

Activity 1 E3 – L1

Job roles for the hair and beauty sector have been provided in the left-hand column. In the right-hand column write down the main person responsible for carrying them out from the list provided. You may use the person responsible more than once.

Job role	Person responsible
Answering the telephone	
Making clients a drink	
Cutting the client's hair using basic techniques	
Carrying out a simple facial	
Preparing the work area	
Organizing the salon	
Taking payments	
Carrying out complex facial treatments	
Carrying out a difficult styling technique	

Person responsible:

Salon manager
Receptionist
Junior stylist
Junior therapist

Junior
Senior therapist
Senior hairdresser

Activity 2 L1

Working on reception

Design a message pad that can be used in the salon to record messages. Make sure you use the following information:

- Who the message is for.
- Who has taken the message.
- The date and time the message was taken.
- What the message is.
- Any action required.
- If the message is urgent.
- How to reply to the message (contact details).

Activity 3 E3 – L1

Using body language

Group activity – Charades

Make two teams. Using the list of words below, team one will mime the actions using different body language. You can use simple props to help you during the mime but you must not speak. Team two will try to identify the word being mimed. Once the second team has correctly identified the mime, change over roles.

List of words

Happy	Anxious	Listening
Sad	Relaxed	Inquisitive
Glad	Defensive	Decisive
Grumpy	Interested	Cold
Angry	Sleepy	Hot
Aggressive	Bored	Flustered

Activity 4 E3 – L1

Design a mood board

Can you find images from magazines or the internet that show different methods of communication? Use the images to design a mood board that you can present to your teacher.

Activity 5 E3 – L1

Calculating client payments

Client	Cost of service or treatment carried out	Answer
Mrs Jones	Has had a hair cut costing £20.00 and a colour costing £22.50. How must does the client need to give you?	
Miss Patel	Has had her nails manicured costing £12.00 and a facial costing £40.50. The client gives you three £20.00 pound notes. How much change will you give her?	
Miss Wong	Has had a manicure costing £18.00 and a pedicure costing £20.00. How much will the bill be? A £3.00 tip is given for the therapist, how much money has the client spent all together?	
Mr Carr	Has been given a bill for £50.00. He has a 10% discount voucher. How much money will he now need to pay?	
Joe	Buys a styling product for his hair. The original price is £8.00. The product has a 25% discount. How much will Joe need to pay?	
Mrs Pantel	Has a facial costing £30.00 and a leg wax costing £8.50. The client gives the receptionist £40.00. How much change will Mrs Pantel receive?	

Activity 6 L1

Working out a simple budget plan using the template below.

In the left-hand column write down all the outgoings that you have to pay for. You can do this on a weekly or monthly basis. In the right-hand column identify how much each of these outgoings costs you.

You will be able to then work out how much money you need to earn to cover your living expenses.

If you have a computer you can use a simple accounting program and record your expenses on an ongoing basis.

Living expenses	Outgoing costs

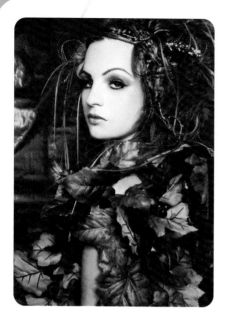

3

Understanding and using colour

There is no blue without yellow and without orange.

VINCENT VAN GOGH, DUTCH ARTIST 1853–1890

In this chapter you are going to learn about:

- Why colour is important for hair and beauty.

- Light and colour theory.

- Primary colours.

- Secondary colours.

- How to create an image using colour – finding inspiration and creating a mood board.

Introduction

The quote above says that there is no blue without yellow and without orange. This is true. Can you imagine a world without colours? How dull would a rainbow look? Colour is very important to everyday life. Uniforms worn at school and for some public service jobs such as the military or nursing are usually dark blue, grey or black, so everyone looks the same. But you can use the colour of your clothes, your make-up, nails and hair to say something about you. You can show how different you are to other people. Some people like to wear very bold, bright colours so that they are noticed in a crowd. Others like to wear plain, dark or neutral colours so that they do not stand out. Colour is also very important for the hair and beauty sector. It is used in all six of the hair and beauty industries – hairdressing, barbering, beauty therapy, nail services, spa therapy and for African type hairdressing and barbering services.

Why colour is important for hair and beauty

The most obvious use is hair colour, make-up and nail polish. But the colour a salon is decorated is also important. And so are the methods that are used to light the rooms in the salon or spa.

Hairdressing and barbering

Colour is used for services in the hairdressing and barbering industries to change the colour of hair. By doing this, hairstyles can look more interesting and a good colour can give hair a glossy, healthy appearance. You can make

IT'S A FACT!

Depth is how light or how dark the hair is. That is, how light the blonde is or how dark the brown is. So, the depth of hair can be light brown, dark blonde, black or the very palest blonde, and everything in between. Hair tone is the colour that you see. So hair can have warm tones such as gold, copper or red. Or hair can have a lack of warmth, which means the tone is ash.

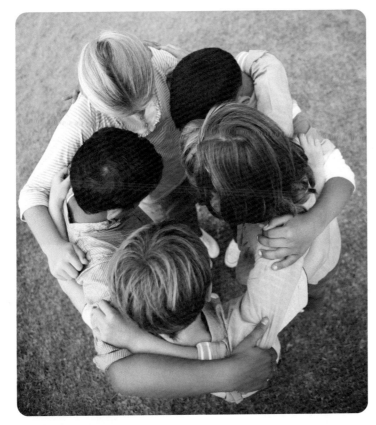

Hair colour can be seen in different depths and tone

WHAT'S NEXT?

When you study hair colouring at Level 2 you will learn lots more about the depth and tones of natural and artificial hair colours. You will also learn about a special code that is used to identify the depth and tone of individual colours. The code is known as the International Colour Chart (ICC). At Level 3 you will learn how to correct hair colour when the colour is not what the client wanted.

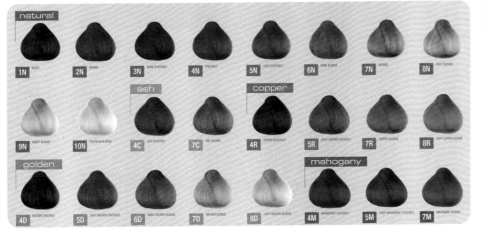

Hair can be coloured in almost every shade you can think of

THE COLOR HERBE® NON-AMMONIA COLOURS. COLOR HERBE® IS THE PROFESSIONAL RANGE OF ANTICA ERBORISTERIA SRL

IT'S A FACT!

The colour of the skin and hair is determined by the amount of a pigment called **melanin** that is found in the skin and hair.

WHAT'S NEXT?

When you study a Level 2 qualification for hair or beauty you will learn more about melanin. You will find out there are different types of melanin. The different types of melanin make skin and hair many different colours.

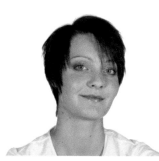

Day make-up

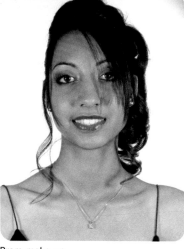

Prom make-up

Make-up is applied for different occasions. The day make-up has much softer colours than the prom make-up

hair lighter or darker. This means you can change the **depth** of the colour. Or you can change the **tone** of the hair by adding warmth, such as red, copper or gold. Or you can add an ash tone, which is a cool colour.

Beauty therapy

Make-up artists will also use colour in the treatments they provide. They apply make-up to clients for a range of different occasions. Before make-up is applied the make-up artist must know what the natural colour and tone of the skin is. Skin colours vary. They can be very dark, almost black or very pale, almost blue, and all shades of brown in-between. Some skin can have golden or olive tones.

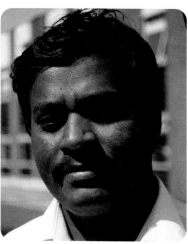

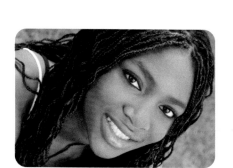

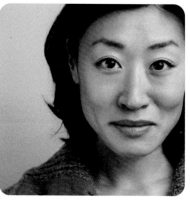

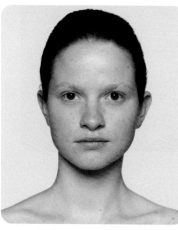

Different racial skin tones are due to the different amounts of melanin in the skin

The make-up artist also needs to know why the make-up is required. Make-up can be required for day time use, for evenings or for photographic purposes. The type of make-up that is applied will depend on the amount of natural light it will be seen in. For example, an evening make-up may be applied using much stronger colours than a day time make-up because it will be seen in low levels of light. Therefore, this will affect the colours that are chosen for the client.

Nail services

Nail technicians will use colour to paint nails and to create nail art. Some colours are used to look natural. For example a French manicure is designed to look like a natural nail. The tips of the nails are painted white and the nail plate in pink or beige. Or nails can be painted in bold, bright colours. Nail art is the creative use of colours. Colours can be painted in stripes, spots or even with miniature pictures drawn on each nail. Some nail art includes the addition of glitter dots, transfers or tapes.

WHAT'S NEXT?

When you are qualified as a nail technician you can enter competitions for nail art and create some amazing designs.

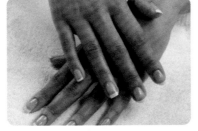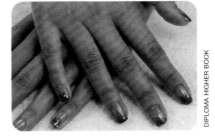

DIPLOMA HIGHER BOOK

Nails can look natural or bright

Spa therapy

Colour is used to light the treatment rooms and waters in salons and spas as a way of reducing stress and providing a feeling of well-being. For example, treatment rooms can be softly lit with shades of violet to calm the nervous system. Lights are used to change the colour of the waters. For example, orange, a warm colour, is used to reduce the effects of depression.

IT'S A FACT!

Treatments using colours are known as **chromotherapy**.

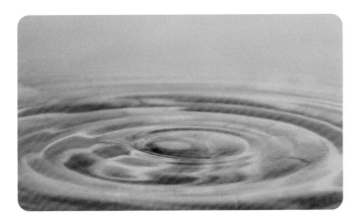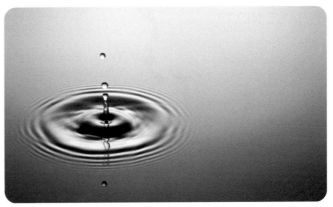

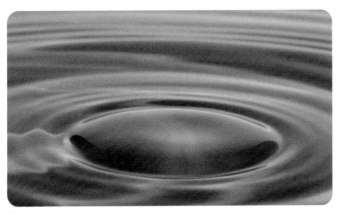

Waters can be lit to enhance well-being

WHAT'S NEXT?

Spa therapists often take additional qualifications to provide treatments that are known as **holistic therapies**. This means therapies that treat the individual as a whole – treating the mind, body and spirit.

Light and colour theory

Colour is a form of light energy. All the colours you see are contained in natural light. Natural light is also referred to as white light. To be able to see the individual colours of the **colour spectrum** the white light needs to be reflected off a flat, polished surface such as glass. If you shine white light through a prism, all the individual colours will separate. The same thing happens when a rainbow is formed. The sun shines through raindrops and the colours of light separate into the colour spectrum.

Natural light is broken by the prism to show the different colours of the colour spectrum

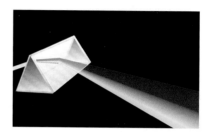

When you look at an object, the actual colour of the object you see is the colour that is reflected. For example, when you see red nail polish, the reason you see red is because all the other colours of the spectrum have been absorbed by the object and only red is reflected. But, even with a red nail polish, you might also see some tones of orange or purple, depending on the other colours that are reflected.

Colours will also vary when seen under different lights. Ordinary electric light bulbs have more red colour and less blue colour than natural daylight. This will make red colour pigments brighter or deeper. Under the same light, blue colour pigments can look darker or blacker.

When salons are planned the lighting is a very important part of the design. Artificial warm, white lights give the nearest match to natural daylight. This is the best type of light to use when colouring hair. Lighting is so important that some hairdressing salons will have a separate colouring area. Any artificial lighting needs to be a close match to natural daylight. The interior of the salon will be also be decorated in a light colour so the surrounding walls do not affect the choice of colour or the appearance of the finished, colour result.

Colour spectrum

You now know that colour is formed through the way objects absorb and reflect different colours within light. When colouring hair, using make-up or applying nail polish the colours used are based on a mixture of pigments found in primary and secondary colours.

Primary colours

A primary colour is a 'pure' colour. This means that it cannot be made by mixing other colours together.

The three **primary colours of pigment** are red, yellow and blue.

Primary colours of pigment

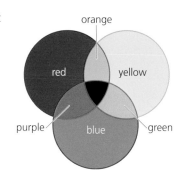

The **primary colours of light** are different to the primary colours of pigment. Light colours are those that come from the sun or from artificial light such as light bulbs. The primary colours of light are red, blue and green.

Primary colours of light

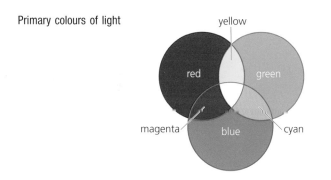

Secondary colours

Secondary colours are made when you mix an equal amount of two primary colours.

So, if you mix an equal amount of:

- Red pigment and yellow pigment = orange.
- Yellow pigment and blue pigment = green.
- Blue pigment and red pigment = purple.

Primary and secondary colours

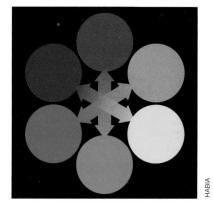

HABIA

The colour wheel shows you all the primary and secondary colours. The colours that are opposite each other are known as **complementary colours**. The colours next to each other are known as **harmonious colours**.

WHAT'S NEXT?

When you study colour in more depth you will learn about a third group of colours that can be made. This group is known as **tertiary colours**.

IT'S A FACT!

Complementary colours are used to neutralize, cancel out or tone down the opposite colour. So, if skin is too red, a green-tinted foundation can be used. If hair is too yellow, a purple-based colour called a **toner** can be used.

WEB LINK

Have a look at this interactive web link. You can click on the buttons to see how colours are grouped together. You will see primary, secondary, harmonious, complementary, warm and cool colours: **www.bbc.co.uk/ schools/gcsebitesize/art/ ao2/elementsrev3.shtml**

SIGNPOST PLTS

Independent enquirer
Reflective learner

ACTIVITY

Prepare yourself with paints of all the primary colours and complete the colour wheel.

1 First colour in the primary colours of pigment.

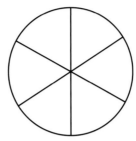

2 To complete the colour wheel, mix an equal amount of two of each primary colour to make the secondary colours.

3 Then see what happens when you mix an equal amount of all the primary and secondary colours together. (Not a very nice colour is it?)

IT'S A FACT!

The most common type of colour blindness is red/green colour blindness.

IT'S A FACT!

Colour blindness affects many more men than women.

Colour blindness

Some people are colour blind. This means that they are unable to see certain colours in the way that others see them. When colouring hair you must be able to see the very small changes in hair colour during the development of the products being used. Some people with certain types of severe colour blindness may not be able to use colouring products and colour hair as part of their job as a hairdresser. This is because they may be unable to detect when a development process is complete and the hair could be damaged.

ACTIVITY

Use the internet and find some more examples like the one on this page of the test images that are used to detect colour blindness.

ACTIVITY

Do you have colour blindness? Look at this image – what can you see?

WEB LINK

Look at this web link: **http://www.etre.com/tools/colourblindsimulator/**. You can upload one of your own photographs and then simulate how colours look to people with different types of colour blindness.

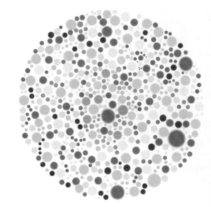

Colour blindness test – can you see the image?

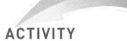

ICT

When you search the internet to find test images for colour blindness you will:

E3 use simple searches to find web-based sources of information

L1 use search techniques to locate and select relevant information.

**SIGNPOST
FUNCTIONAL
SKILL**

ICT

When you look at the web link to simulate colour blindness you will interact with ICT for a given purpose and you will be able to recognize and use interface features and insert media. **E3 – L1**

**SIGNPOST
FUNCTIONAL
SKILL**

Creating a themed image using colour

The hair and beauty industries are all about image. The results from many of the treatments and services are very visual. For example, if you colour or style your hair in a new way, all your friends will notice. Make-up can be natural or can be very bright and adventurous. You have different effects for different occasions. Nail art is amazing. The effects that you can create and the colours that you can use are only limited by your imagination.

Image themes

Hair stylists, make-up artists and nail technicians can all create images. The images can be used in magazines, on catwalks, in television and movies. Or they can be just what the client has requested.

To create a themed image that might be used in a magazine, or in a competition, you first need to have some ideas of what you want your finished image to look like. You need a theme. You can find inspiration by looking all around you, from your environment, films, television, books and magazines.

You might like to create an image because you have been inspired by something you have seen:

- In movies.
- In nature.
- In your local environment.
- During the changing of the seasons.
- When listening to music.
- When learning about different traditional cultures and folklore.
- Something from another period of history.
- When you have travelled to other countries.

Creating a mood board

Once you have found your inspiration you can link your theme to a look you want to create by making a **mood board**.

A mood board is a collection of items that are gathered together and based on your theme. The mood board will show you, and other people, what inspires you when planning to create your image. For example, you might want to create a hairstyle, make-up or nail art that has the theme of 'autumn'. You might have been inspired by the colours of gold, yellow, brown and copper and you might want the hair, make-up or nails to include these colours.

So, you would make a mood board made up of these colours and images of autumn. The mood board might have fabrics, lace, ribbons, buttons, examples of hair, make-up or nail art that has been completed using the colours of autumn. You could also include your thoughts and ideas written on pieces of paper. The mood board does not have to be neat. You can even tear pictures out of a magazine and stick them straight onto your mood board. The mood board should, in one glance, tell another person what your ideas are.

Method for making a mood board Include some or all of the following on your mood board:

1 Look through magazines and find examples of the things that are inspiring you to create your image. Cut or tear out the images.

2 Find examples of the type of finished look you might want to create.

3 Find examples of fabrics in the colours that inspire you.

4 Apply example colours of make-up or nail polish to pieces of paper. The colours will be those that you want to use when you create your image.

5 If you are going to create a hairstyle, find some samples of hair swatches from colour charts, or colour swatches of hair to apply to your mood

TOP TIP

Remember, you can include *anything* on your mood board that inspires you. And, it does not have to be neatly presented – it should be creative.

Example of a mood board used to inspire an image based on the theme 'Autumn'

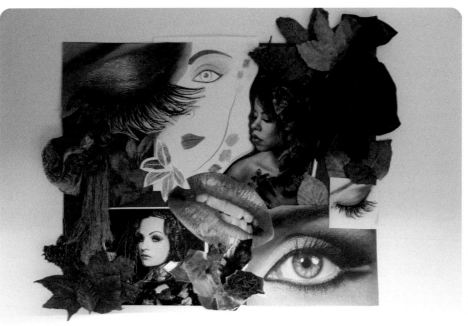

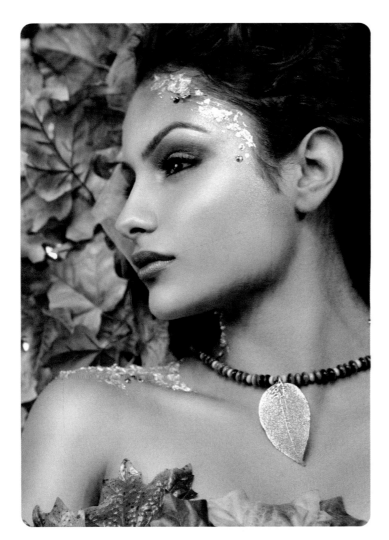

The finished 'Autumn' look

board. The hair swatches should be similar to the hair colour on the model you will use to create your image.

6 Stick or pin the items you have found to your mood board.

ACTIVITY

Make a mood board for a theme that has inspired you. Then create an image on a model to reflect the mood board. The image you create can be for hairstyling, make-up for any occasion, or nail art. Present your mood board to other people in your class. Tell them about your mood board and the inspiration behind the theme. When you have created your image on your model, think about what you did really well. Did the mood board influence the end result? Think about what you might do better if you created the image again. You could hold a competition and ask a teacher from another class to judge the mood boards and the final, created image on your models.

SIGNPOST PLTS

Independent enquirer
Creative thinker
Self-manager
Reflective learner

What you have learnt

Why colour is important for hair and beauty:

- Colour is used for many of the hair and beauty industry treatments and services.
- The lighting and the decoration of salons and spas is very important for colour application and use.

Light and colour theory:

- Colour is a form of light energy.
- All colours you see are contained in white light.
- The individual colours are known as a colour spectrum.
- The colour of an object is determined by the colour that is reflected.

Primary colours:

- The primary colours of pigment are red, yellow and blue.
- The primary colours of light are red, blue and green.
- Primary colours are 'pure' colours. They cannot be made by mixing other colours together.

Secondary colours:

- Secondary colours are made by mixing equal amounts of two of the primary colours together.

How to create an image using colour – finding inspiration and creating a mood board:

- Stylists, make-up artists and nail technicians can all create images with the skills they have. The images can be created for magazines, television, film, catwalks or even for competitions.
- To create an image, you need a theme.
- You can create mood board to illustrate the things that inspire you for creating an image.

ASSESSMENT ACTIVITIES

Activity 1 E3 – L1

These are short answer questions. Read the question carefully. When you have finished, write down your answer.

Q1 Colour is not used for treatments in the spa industry – is this question true or false?

Q2 Give one example of how colour can be used in the hairdressing industry.

Q3 Give one example of how colour can be used by a nail technician.

Q4 How many individual colours make up the colour spectrum?

Q5 State the reason why you can see that a nail polish is red.

Q6 State the three primary colours of pigment.

Q7 State the three primary colours of light.

Q8 Which colours would you mix to make green?

Q9 State why you would use a mood board.

Q10 Give two sources of inspiration for creating an image.

Activity 2 E1 – L1

Four in a Row

Work with a partner or split into two teams. Answer the following questions with 'True' or 'False'. If you are correct, colour in one of the squares. The winner is the first to get four squares in a row. They can be horizontal, vertical or diagonal. If you can see your partner or the other team getting close to four squares you can block them.

True or false questions

1 Colour is used in all the hair and beauty industries.

2 Colouring hair makes it look dull.

3 The tone of hair means how light or dark the hair is.

4 An example of a warm tone used when colouring hair is copper.

5 Before a make-up artist applies make-up they need to know what colour the client's hair is.

6 Melanin is only found in skin.

7 Stronger colours can be used for day make-up as it is seen in natural light.

8 Gold is an example of a cool tone that is used when colouring hair.

9 A French manicure is used to make the nails look bright and bold.

10 Spa treatments that use colours for improving well-being are known as chromotherapy.

11 Red is an example of a warm tone that is used when colouring hair.

12 Colour is a form of heat energy.

13 The colour spectrum is made of six separate colours.

14 If the skin is too red, the colour can be toned down by using a green-coloured foundation.

15 To see the colours of a spectrum you can shine black light through a prism.

16 The colours in the colour spectrum are never formed in the same order.

17 Make-up applied for a daytime look should not look the same as make-up applied for an evening event.

18 When creating nail art you can use spots and stripes.

19 Ordinary electric light bulbs have more red and less blue colour than natural daylight.

20 A room used for colouring hair in a salon will be painted in dark colours.

21 Colour can be used to reduce stress.

22 Harmonious colours are next to each other on the colour wheel.

23 Yellow is a pure colour of pigment.

24 If you mix red and yellow you will make orange.

25 Colours next to each other in the colour circle are known as complementary colours.

26 Mixing blue and red will make green.

27 The primary colours of light are red, yellow and blue.

28 An example of a cool colour is blue.

29 You can see all the colours of the spectrum on a colour wheel.

30 If the end result of a colour on hair is too yellow, a green-coloured toner can be used.

31 Flattering colours are used to neutralize, or cancel out the opposite colour.

32 A mood board will show others what has inspired you.

33 To make a secondary colour you have to mix equal amounts of two primary colours.

34 Hairdressers do not create images.

35 You can be inspired to create an image by looking at your environment.

36 When creating a mood board you can use torn-out images from magazines.

4

Skincare, make-up and face painting

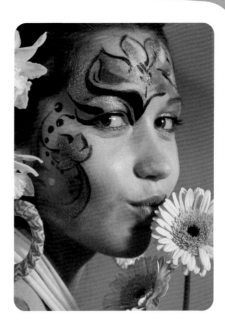

Beauty is in the eye of the beholder.

ANON.

In this chapter you are going to learn about:

- Importance of good skincare.

- Basic structure and function of the skin.

- Bone structure.

- Preparing the work area and tools, products and equipment for make-up application.

- Preparing and carrying out a basic skincare treatment.

- Factors that affect the choice of make-up products.

- Preparing for and carrying out basic make-up techniques.

- Preparing for and carrying out face painting design.

- Removal of make-up products.

Introduction

The world of skincare and make-up can be glamorous and exciting. There are so many different looks that you can create when using make-up, from natural beauty to glamorous, glittering diva.

Looking after your skin is the foundation to looking good. You can then use make-up to enhance your natural features or help change your image. As a beauty therapist you can make someone feel and look better from the skincare and make-up treatments that you carry out in the salon.

In this chapter you will learn about the skills and knowledge needed to understand how to look after the skin, you will learn about bone structure, the skin's structure and its characteristics, and how to carry out a skincare routine and apply make-up. You will also learn how to create simple face painting designs.

Importance of good skincare

The way you live your life can be reflected in the way that your skin looks. You can't have an unhealthy diet, eat fried food and drink fizzy drinks, stay up late at night and still expect your skin to be clear and glowing.

Not only do you need to look after your skin by eating a healthy diet but you also need to make sure it is really clean and moisturized. Every day dirt, sweat and make-up can build up on the surface of your skin and block pores. This can lead to skin problems, especially if you do not have a good skincare routine.

IT'S A FACT!

Your skin can be affected by many things, which could include:

Poor nutrients	Smoking	Alcohol	Medication/drugs
Stress	Hormonal changes	Extreme weather	Sunburn
Central heating	Illness	Poor skincare	Lack of fresh air

A simple but effective skincare routine is best, so that you can easily fit it into your everyday hygiene habits. It should be as easy as brushing your teeth, and like brushing your teeth it should be done twice a day to get the best results.

Clear and glowing skin is very attractive

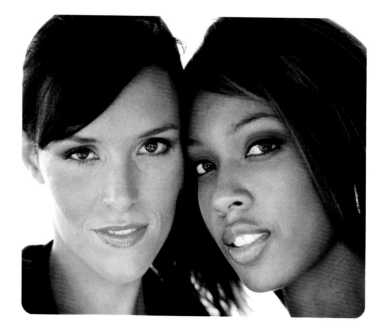

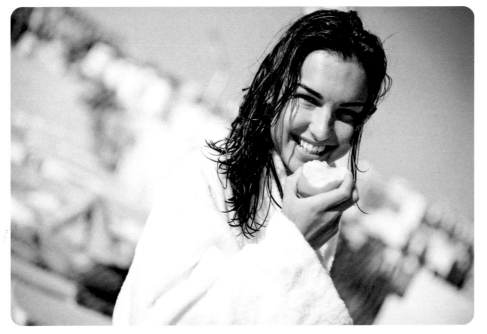

Healthy eating reflects in your skin

The basic structure of the skin

The skin is the largest organ of the body. The appearance of the skin varies. For example, the skin of a child looks different to that of an adult. The skin of a young person will be soft and smooth, but as you get older the skin becomes thinner and loses its elasticity. You will notice that, with aging, the skin becomes dryer and develops wrinkles.

The condition of the skin will also vary. Some people have very dry skin, others have oily skin. Excessively oily skins can sometimes be a problem at

IT'S A FACT!

The function of melanin is to protect the skin from the harmful ultraviolet rays of the sun.

IT'S A FACT!

Melanin is the colour pigment in skin and hair and the iris of the eye.

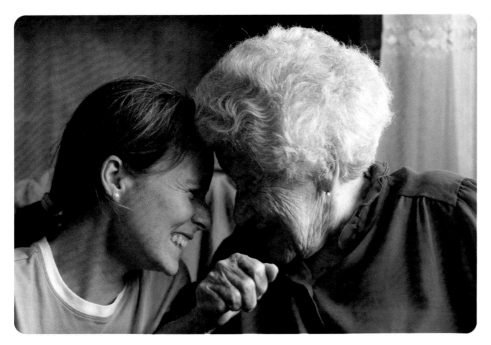

Young and old skin

WHAT'S NEXT?

When you study the skin as part of a Level 2 hair or beauty qualification, you will learn all the names of the five layers of the epidermis. The layers, from the bottom to the top, are known as stratum germinativum, stratum spinosum, stratum granulosum, stratum lucidum and stratum corneum.

IT'S A FACT!

Stratum means 'layer'.

WWW

WEB LINK

Try this interactive web link. Label the skin diagram and answer some questions. You can play drag and drop activities in a quiz about the structure of skin. **http://www.abpischools.org .uk/page/modules/skin/skin5 .cfm**

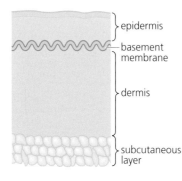

Layers of the skin

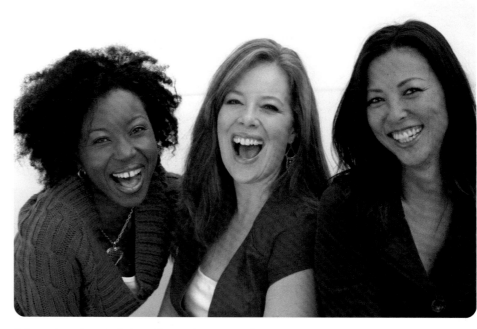

Skin can be pale or dark depending on the amount of melanin present

puberty. During this time you may notice more sebum is produced and the skin can become spotty.

The colour of the skin changes depending on the amount of melanin, the natural colour pigment, that is present. People with black skin have more melanin than those with pale skin.

The layers of the skin

The skin is made up of three layers. The top layer is called the **epidermis**. This is the layer of skin that you can see and touch. The epidermis itself has five layers. New skin cells are continuously produced in the bottom of the epidermis. The skin cells then rise to the surface and as they do become flatter. By the time they reach the very top, the cells are dead and flake off.

The second layer of the skin is called the **dermis**. This is an important layer as it contains all the appendages of the skin.

The third layer of the skin is called the **subcutaneous layer**. This layer contains fat cells which give your body and face its shape and form.

SIGNPOST FUNCTIONAL SKILL

ICT

When you look at the web link for the skin structure you will interact with ICT for a given purpose and you will be able to recognize and use interface features. **E3** and **L1**

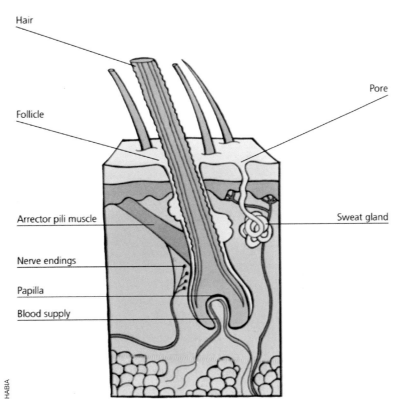

Hair

Follicle

Arrector pili muscle

Nerve endings

Papilla

Blood supply

Pore

Sweat gland

Cross-section of the skin structure

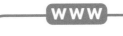

WHAT'S NEXT?

When you study the skin as part of a Level 2 hair or beauty qualification, you will learn about the appendages of the skin in greater detail.

WWW
WEB LINK

Look at this web link. You can see an animation showing the skin cells of the epidermis developing, and rising to the top layer before flaking away. http://www.abpischools.org.uk/page/modules/skin/skin2.cfm?coSiteNavigation_allTopic=1

The functions of the skin

Your skin has lots of functions. It is there to:

- Protect you – protection.
- Take in vitamins – absorption.
- Get rid of waste products – excretion and secretion.
- Control your temperature – temperature control.
- Help you to feel things – sense of touch.

Protection

The skin helps to protect you in lots of ways:

- The barrier of skin protects your organs from invading germs.
- The coating of the natural oil (**sebum**) and sweat creates another protective layer against germs called the **acid mantle**.
- The nerve endings in the skin mean that you can tell if something is too hot or too cold to touch. Or you can tell if something is sharp and likely to hurt you.

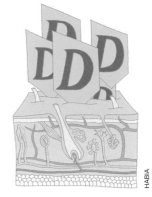

Skin function – protection

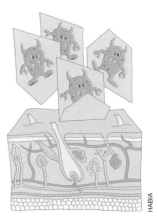

Skin function – absorption

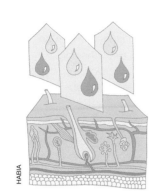

Skin function – excretion and secretion

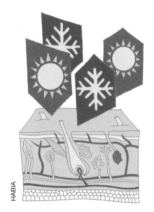

Skin function – temperature control

SIGNPOST PLTS

Teamworker

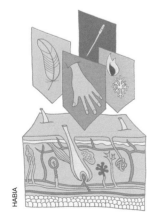

Skin function – sense of touch

Absorption

Although the skin acts as a barrier, it also allows certain things to pass through. One important vitamin, Vitamin D, is absorbed by the skin. Vitamin D is needed to help develop healthy bones.

Excretion and secretion

When you get too hot your body produces sweat. The sweat helps to cool the skin as it evaporates. Your body also excretes sebum, the natural oil of the skin. The sebum helps to moisturize the skin, stopping it from becoming too dry.

Temperature control

It is your blood supply that helps you control your body temperature. You need to keep your body temperature at the correct level so that your organs can all work properly. Normal body temperature is 36.8°C or 98.6°F. If you are too hot your blood vessels become wider to help to cool you down. This is why you might look very red! If you are too cold, the blood vessels become narrower to help reduce lost heat. This is why you might look pale, even blue, when cold! You may also shiver and this helps to keep you warm. The arrector pili muscle will also make your hair stand on end to trap warm air near the body – and this causes goose bumps.

Sense of touch

In the dermis of skin there are many nerve endings. The nerve endings help you to sense different things. Some nerve endings near the surface of the skin allow you to feel the lightest of touches. Others that lie deeper in the skin allow you to feel heavier touches, or pain. The nerve endings also tell you if something is hot or cold to touch.

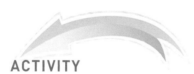

ACTIVITY

You can see the effects of touch by touching the skin on the back of the hand or the arm with a metal, two-pronged roller or hair pin. First, bend the ends of the roller or hair pin and separate them so they are five cm apart. Then, working with a partner, ask them to close their eyes while you touch different areas on the back of their hand or arm. Ask your partner to say how many points they can feel on their skin – one or two? You will find out that areas of the skin with more nerve endings will allow you to feel two points. Where there are fewer nerve endings, you will only feel one point – even though you have used two.

Bone structure

Did you know that the bones and muscles of the head and face determine the shape of our head and face and our individual features? Hair and beauty professionals need to know the position of bones and muscles so that they can enhance a client's good features and help hide other features. This is particularly important for example when you are applying make-up.

Bones of the head and face

The **skull** is made up of the bones that form the head, this is also known as the **cranium** and the face. The cranium is the large bony casing that surrounds your brain; it will protect it from bumps and knocks. Your cranium is made up of eight large flat bones that are fixed together by joints called **sutures**.

There are 14 bones of the face:

- Two bones that make up the eye socket.
- Seven bones that make up the nose.
- Two bones that make up the upper jaw.
- One bone that makes up the lower jaw.
- Two bones that make up the check bones.

Apart from a bone in your nose and your lower jaw bone, all your facial bones come in pairs, one on each side of your face. That's why your face is **symmetrical**.

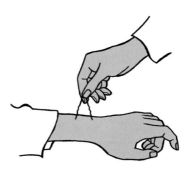
Experiment to illustrate the sense of touch

IT'S A FACT!

The skull is made up of 22 bones. There are 14 bones of the face and eight bones of the head.

WHAT'S NEXT?

When you study the bones of the cranium as part of a Level 2 hair or beauty qualification, you will learn the full names of the eight head bones and where they are located.

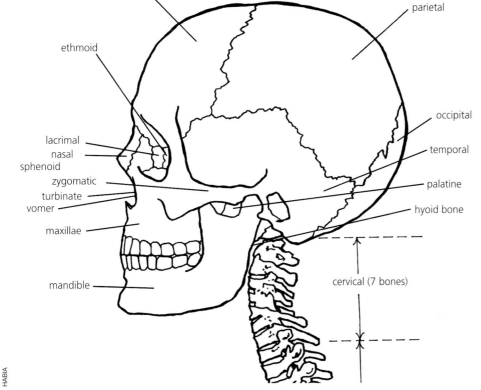
Bones of the skull

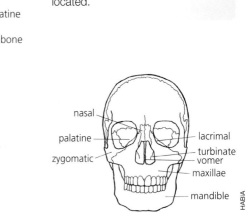
Bones of the face

ACTIVITY

Why not find out a bit more about the bones of the head and face. Use the internet to look for more information. You can try the websites listed below:

http://home.comcast.net/~wnor/lesson1.htm
http://www.ivy-rose.co.uk/HumanBody/Skeletal/Bones_CranialandFacial.php
http://www.bbc.co.uk/science/humanbody/body/factfiles/skull/frontal_in_skull.shtml

SIGNPOST PLTS

Independent enquirer

**SIGNPOST
FUNCTIONAL
SKILLS**

ICT

When you are looking at websites for information on bones of the head and face you will interact with ICT for a given purpose and you will be able to recognize and use interface features. **E3** and **L1**

IT'S A FACT!

The lower jawbone is the only bone of the skull that can move. All the other bones are joined together to make it rigid.

WHAT'S NEXT?

When you study the bones of the face as part of a Level 2 hair or beauty qualification, you will learn the full names of the 14 bones and were they are located.

IT'S A FACT!

Muscles are very clever structures; they are long lasting, self-healing and have the ability to get stronger when you exercise.

Muscles

Muscles cover the whole skeleton of our body; we need muscles to be able to move about. The muscles of the head and face are all very small. When a muscle moves, it also moves the facial skin; this creates all our different facial expressions such as frowning or smiling.

WHAT'S NEXT?

When you progress to Level 2 beauty therapy you will learn a lot more about bone structure and the function that bones and muscles have, not only on the head and face but on the whole body.

Skin types

The way to have lovely looking skin is to understand your skin type. As a beauty therapist you will have to learn all about skin type and how to recognize your client's skin type. You will need this information so that you can choose and use the right products for your client.

There are four main skin types:

- Normal.
- Dry.
- Greasy/oily.
- Combination.

Knowing how to recognize different skin types and then using the correct products will help the skin to look and feel good.

Skin conditions

Before you begin any type of treatment as a professional beauty therapist you will need to examine your client's skin. You need to do this to identify the skin type and also to identify if there is a skin condition that might mean the client cannot have a facial treatment. This is called a skin analysis and you will do this as part of the consultation with your client.

Different types of skin condition display different symptoms from redness, cracking skin and weeping fluid, to spots and scabs.

ACTIVITY

With a partner or on your own, work out which skin type you are by circling a, b or c to the following questions that you think best describes your skin.

When you look into a mirror does your skin:

a Look healthy with even skin colour?

b Have an uneven colour, do you have any freckles?

c Look pale, sallow or shiny?

When you touch your skin:

a Does it feel firm and smooth?

b Can you feel small hard spots or lumps around the upper part of your face or does it feel dry and flaky in some areas?

c Does it feel moist or slippery to touch?

Does your skin:

a Rarely get spots?

b Become red and irritated particularly when you use certain products or when you are in different environmental conditions, e.g. cold or hot weather?

c Frequently get spots?

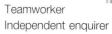

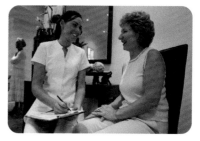

Client consultation

Results

Mainly a – you may have a normal skin type

Mainly b – you may have a dry skin type

Mainly c – you may have a greasy/oily skin type

Mixture of b and c – you may have a combination skin type.

Combination skin has both oily and dry areas usually in a T-zone. The T-zone goes across the forehead and down the nose and chin. This area is oily. The cheeks are usually dry.

Skin conditions can be grouped in to four main types:

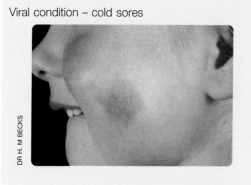

Viral condition – cold sores

DR H. M BECKS

Viral conditions: Groups of very simple organisms that are smaller than bacteria and can cause infections and disease.

Bacterial condition – impetigo

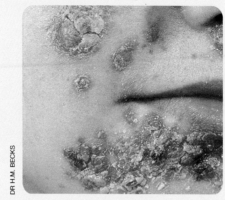

DR H.M. BECKS

Bacterial conditions: Bacteria are a large group of micro-organisms that can also cause infection and disease.

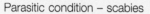

Parasitic condition – scabies

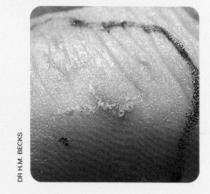

DR H.M. BECKS

Parasitic conditions: When an animal or plant lives in or on our body so that it can feed from it.

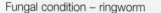

WHAT'S NEXT?

When you progress to Level 2 you will learn all about the different skin types and conditions and how to recognize them. This will be important, as it will affect your decisions during the consultation process with your client.

Fungal condition – ringworm

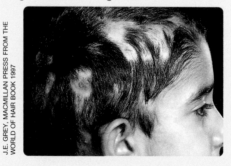

J.E. GREY, MACMILLAN PRESS FROM THE WORLD OF HAIR BOOK 1997

Fungal conditions: Fungi are microscopic plants that do not have leaves or roots. Fungal infections live off the waste products produced by our skin.

Preparing the work area for a facial treatment

When preparing your work area for a facial treatment for a client, you need to make sure that the environment is comfortable and that the room is ready with all the tools, materials, equipment and products you may need.

For the treatment room you will need to make sure:

- The temperature is nice and warm, but not too stuffy.
- The lighting is soft and not too bright, so that your client feels relaxed.
- The background music is not too loud.
- Any fragrant candles being used to make the client more relaxed are safely placed out the way.

When carrying out a facial treatment you will also need to make sure that the treatment room has the following specialist equipment:

A facial treatment couch

Treatment bed/couch or chair: For the client to relax on while the treatment is being carried out.

HABIA AND CENGAGE LEARNING

Equipment trolley

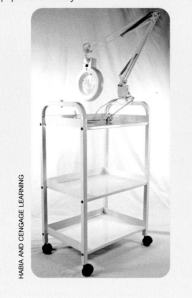

Equipment trolley: To hold the equipment, tools, materials and products that you will need to use during the treatment.

HABIA AND CENGAGE LEARNING

Beauty chair

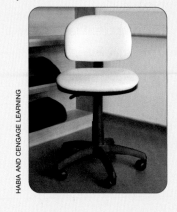

HABIA AND CENGAGE LEARNING

Beauty stool/chair: A specially designed chair/stool that you can sit on during a beauty treatment.

When preparing your equipment, tools and materials you will need to make sure you have the following items ready in the room:

- Blankets/duvet/linen: Clean bedding to keep your client warm during the treatment.

- Towels: These must be clean and soft.

- Gown/bathrobe: A clean gown is used to protect the client's modesty. Lined swing waste bin: For disposing of waste materials.

- Sterilizer: For sterilizing your tools, to prevent the spread of infection.

On your equipment trolley you will need to make sure you have the following items:

- Spatulas: Clean spatulas, used to remove product from jars or containers.

- Bowls: A selection of different-sized bowls, for storing cotton wool, water and for your client's jewellery.

- Headband: To protect and keep your client's hair out of the way from facial products as you work.

- Sponges: Sterilized sponges to remove the face mask product from your client's skin.

- Cotton wool (dry and damp): To use during the treatment.

- Cotton buds: To remove any make-up close to the eyelashes.

- Tissues: Used during the treatment.

- Mask brush: Used to apply a mask product to your client's face and neck.

- Hand mirror: You will use this as part of the consultation with your client at the beginning and end of the facial treatment.

- Facial skincare products: These will include:

  ○ Eye make-up remover.

  ○ Skin cleanser.

  ○ Skin toner.

○ Moisturizer.

○ Facial scrub.

○ Face mask.

Skincare products

Skincare product	Different types of facial products available
Cleanser	Cleansers are used to remove dirt and make-up from the skin. ● Cleaning lotion: A strong **astringent**-type cleanser that is more effective for oily and congested skins. ● Cleansing milk: A gentle cleaner that is effective on young skin but may be drying on mature skins. ● Cleansing cream: A heavier cleanser, more effective on dry and more mature skins. ● Foaming cleanser: Effective on combination and oily skin types.
Toner	Toners refresh the skin and remove any remains of cleanser. They are designed to tighten the pores of the skin. ● Fresheners: Very mild, best for dry and mature skins. ● Toners: Slightly stronger than fresheners with a mild astringent effect, most effective on normal skin types. ● Astringent: Very strong as it contains alcohol and sometimes **antiseptic**. Best for combination and oily skin types.
Moisturizer	Moisturizers are used to prevent the skin from drying out and protect the skin from the environment such as the wind, sun or central heating. ● Moisturizing lotion: A lighter product best used on young and oily skin types. ● Moisturizing mousse: A lighter 'whipped' cream ideal for normal skin types. ● Moisturizing cream: A heavier and richer cream ideal for dry and mature skin types.

COURTESY OF GUINOT

Skincare product

Different types of facial products available

Facial scrub

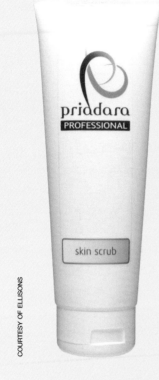

COURTESY OF ELLISONS

Facial masks are designed to remove dead skin cells and help make the skin appear brighter, cleaner and glowing.

Most facial scrubs consist of a cream that contains fine particles that are abrasive and so remove the dead skin cells.

Face mask

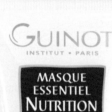

COURTESY OF ELLISONS

Face masks are designed to give a more concentrated effect on certain skin types and conditions. They reinforce the effects of cleaning, or help improve the moisture content of the skin.

There are two types of masks:

- Setting masks: These set on to the skin causing a tightening sensation.
- Non-setting masks: These masks do not set when applied to the skin and are the most popular type to use in the salon.

Carrying out a basic skincare treatment

Once you have organized your equipment trolley with all the tools, products and materials you will need to carry out a facial treatment, and then prepared your client and yourself, you are ready to start the treatment.

There are five basic steps.

Step 1: Cleansing

Cleansing is one of the most important stages in the facial treatment. It removes the dirt and any make-up from the skin's surface.

There are two parts to cleansing:

1 Superficial cleansing to remove make-up and surface grease and dirt.

2 Deep cleansing to give a deeper cleanse to the face, to remove every trace of dirt and ensure the skin is squeaky clean.

Superficial cleansing The procedure for superficial cleansing is:

- Eyes and lashes.
- Lips.
- Face and neck.

Follow the step-by-step pictures to see how it is done:

Step-by-step superficial cleansing

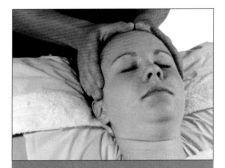

1 Wash your hands, and dry thoroughly. Apply pressure to the scalp, to start the relaxation process. Ensure the headband is firmly in place to protect the hair.

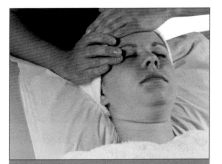

2 Cleanse each eye separately. Start with the right eye, apply eye make-up remover in small circular movements over the eyelid and lashes. Ensure the pressure is very light. Always support the eyebrow area with your free hand. Repeat on the left eye.

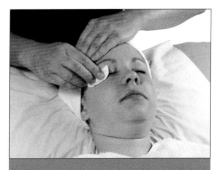

3 Take damp cotton wool pads and stroke the pads down over the lid and lashes, until all the eye make-up has been removed.

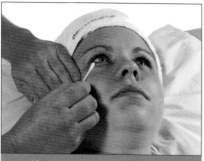

4 If necessary use a cotton bud to get the last traces of eye shadow and mascara off.

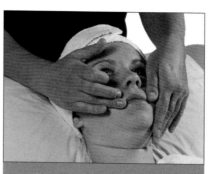

5 Cleanse each side of the lips separately. Apply a cleaning lotion or milk in small circles to the right side of the mouth, supporting the corner of the mouth with your free hand.

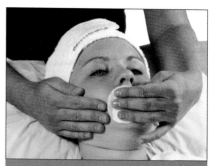

6 Take damp cotton wool pads, and stroke inwards across the lips to remove all lipstick, repeat until the lips are clean.

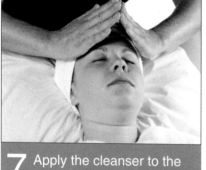

7 Apply the cleanser to the face and start at the forehead with light strokes.

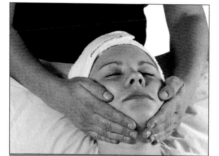

8 Work slowly onto the cheeks, with circular movements, finish on the neck area with sliding movements.

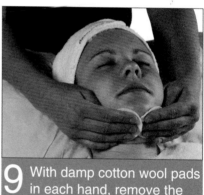

9 With damp cotton wool pads in each hand, remove the cleanser with light upward strokes. Facial sponges can also be used to remove the cleanser. Repeat until all the cleanser is removed.

Deep cleansing The deep cleansing procedure involves a routine of 10 massage movements to help the cleansing product to be absorbed deep into the skin's pores and ensure the skin is cleaned thoroughly.

Apply your cleanser to both of your hands and then apply to your client's face and neck in long flowing strokes. Then follow the next set of step-by-step pictures; it should take about 10 minutes to go through the massage strokes:

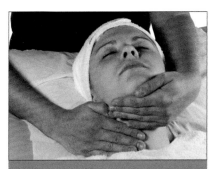

1 Stroking (neck area) – using your fingertips stroke up both sides of the neck, then outward under the jaw, and back down lightly to the starting position.

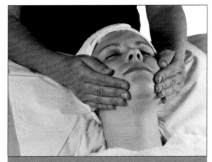

2 Finger kneading to the chin area.

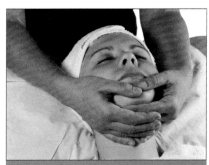

3 Thumb kneading to the entire chin area.

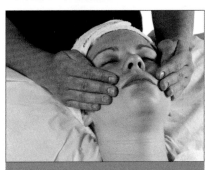

4 Circling (cheek area) – apply small circles with fingertips to entire cheek area, starting at the chin, working up around the nose, across the cheek bone and back along lower cheek to chin.

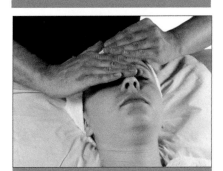

5 Gliding (nose) – with ring and middle fingers of right hand, start at base of nose and glide along the length of the nose and off the end, followed by the left hand.

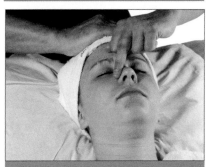

6 Circling (eye area) – with the middle finger circle around each eye. Start on the inner eyebrow, stroke out along brow bone and inwards under the eye. Adapt to form a 'figure of 8' movement, with each hand working alternately.

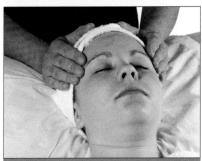

7 Circling (forehead) – with ring and middle fingers perform small circles across the forehead.

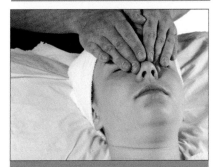

8 Sliding (eye area) – with index, middle and ring fingers, slide outwards around the brow bone and underneath the eye area. At the end of the stroke, lift and apply pressure with each individual finger on the brow bone.

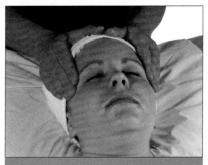

9 Circling (temple area) – with the index, middle and ring fingers circle on the temple area, applying slight pressure. Pause at the end, and hold for a count of three.

Once you have completed Step 1, the cleansing process, you can then follow the remaining four steps:

- Step 2: Application and removal of a facial scrub.
- Step 3: Application and removal of a face mask.
- Step 4: Application of a toner.
- Step 5: Application of a moisturizer.

Step 2: Facial scrub

Application and removal of a facial scrub

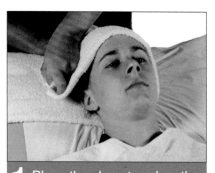

1 Place the clean towel on the pillow, and wrap the towel carefully over the head, protecting the hairline.

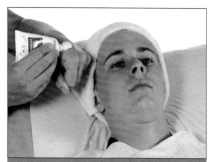

2 Choose the appropriate scrub for the skin type. Always read and follow the manufacturer's instructions carefully. Place a small amount of scrub on the back of your hand.

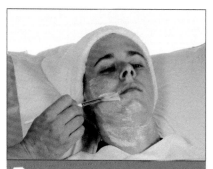

3 Apply the scrub to the face with a mask brush. Explain to the client the sensation they will feel.

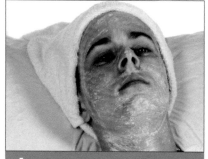

4 Make sure the scrub is applied evenly all over the neck, chin, cheeks, nose and forehead.

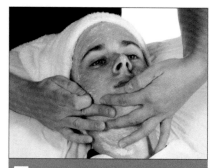

5 With small circular motions, lightly massage the entire face and neck in an upwards direction. Be careful on delicate areas such as the cheeks and avoid the eye area and lips. If the scrub dries out too much, and starts to drag, add water by dampening your hands.

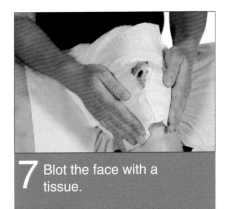

6 The scrub is left on the skin for the recommended time, according to the manufacturer's instructions. Use warm damp sponges to remove the scrub, starting at the neck, make sure you check the hairline and around the nostrils. Do not have the sponges too wet or it will be uncomfortable for the client.

7 Blot the face with a tissue.

Step 3: Face mask

Application and removal of a setting facial mask

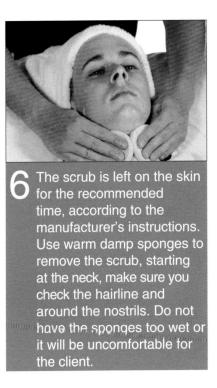

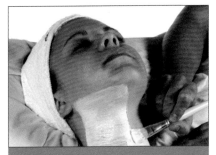

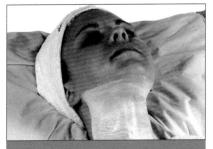

1 Choose the appropriate mask for the skin type. Always read and follow the manufacturer's instructions carefully. Apply a small amount of mask to the back of your hand.

2 Using a clean mask brush, apply the mask quickly so the skin gets the maximum effect from the active ingredients in the mask. Start at the base of the neck.

3 It is important to apply the mask quickly and evenly so it doesn't dry out sooner in some parts of the face or neck, as it could irritate the skin. Explain to the client the sensation they will feel.

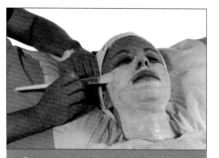

4 Work quickly and carefully upwards, avoid the lips, nostrils, eye area and eyebrows.

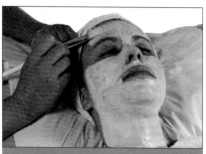

5 Finish on the forehead, being careful to avoid the hairline.

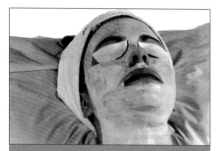

6 Dampened cotton wool pads are applied to the eyes, this helps to relax the client. The mask is left on the skin for the recommended time, according to the anufacturer's instructions.

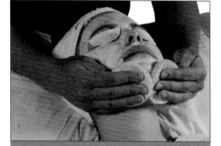

7 Use warm damp sponges to remove the mask, starting on the neck area. Do not forget to remove the eye pads and continue on to the cheek area. Do not have the sponges too wet or it will be uncomfortable for the client.

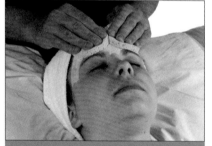

8 Be careful to remove every last trace of the mask, which can be a challenge with a 'setting' mask.

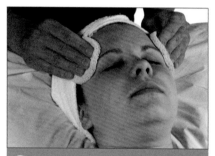

9 Check the hairline, around the nostrils and under the chin to ensure there are no traces of mask left on the skin.

Application and removal of a non-setting mask

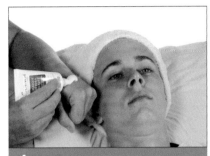

1 Choose the appropriate mask for the skin type. Always read and follow the manufacturer's instructions carefully. Apply a small amount of mask to the back of your hand.

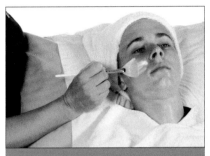

2 Using a clean mask brush, apply the mask quickly so the skin gets the maximum effect from the active ingredients in the mask. Start at the base of the neck and work carefully upwards, finishing on the forehead. Avoid the lips, nostrils, eye area, eyebrows and hairline. Apply the mask evenly so it doesn't dry out earlier in some parts of the face or neck. Explain to the client the sensation they will feel.

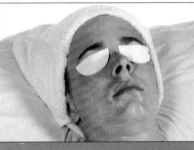

3 Dampened cotton wool pads are applied to the eyes, this helps to relax the client. The mask is left on the skin for the recommended time, according to the manufacturer's instructions.

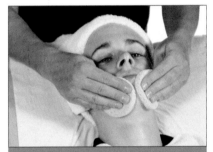

4 Remove the eye pads, and use warm damp sponges to remove the mask. Do not have the sponges too wet or it will be uncomfortable for the client. Be careful to remove every last trace of the mask, which can be a challenge, check the hairline, around the nostrils and under the chin.

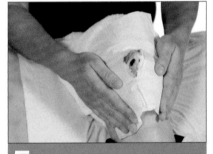

5 Blot the face with a tissue.

Step 4: Toning

Application of a toner

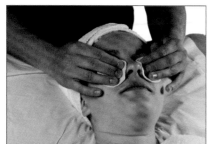

1 Choose the appropriate toner for the skin type. Apply the toner to two damp cotton wool pads. Starting at the base of the neck, wipe the pads gently over the neck and face using long sweeping, flowing strokes.

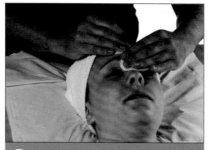

2 Continue over the entire face.

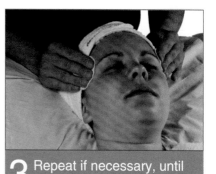

3 Repeat if necessary, until the skin is free of grease or product.

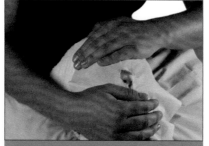

4 Blot the skin to remove any excess toner. Take a facial tissue, tear a small hole in the middle for the nose, apply to the face, and gently press all over to absorb any excess toner.

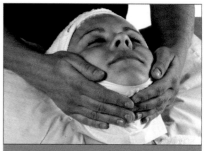

5 Remove the tissue, fold in half and apply to the neck area, and gently press.

Step 5: Moisturizing

Application of a moisturizer

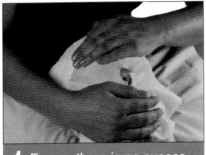

1 Ensure there is no excess toner on the skin, and that a tissue has been used to blot the face and neck.

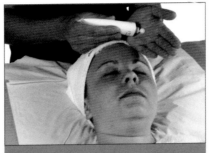

2 Choose the correct moisturizer for the skin type.

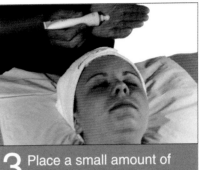

3 Place a small amount of moisturizer in the palm of your hand.

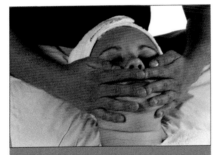

4 Apply the moisturizer sparingly to the neck, chin, cheeks, nose and forehead.

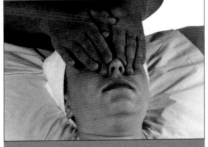

5 Lightly massage the moisturizer into the face and neck with upwards and outwards flowing strokes.

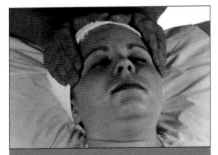

6 End with light pressure on the temples.

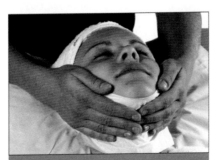

7 If necessary use a tissue to blot any excess moisturizer.

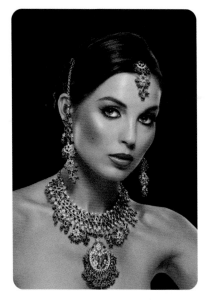

Make-up effects

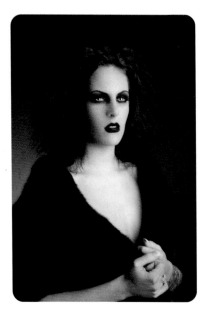

Make-up effects

Make-up

Make-up gives you the ability to be creative, to be whoever you want to be … a girl-next-door look, like Jennifer Aniston? Or a more glamorous diva, like Beyonce?

Make-up gives us the ability to create whatever look you or your client wants.

Make-up can be used for a variety of reasons:

- To enhance natural features.
- To disguise or soften natural features.
- To conceal spots and blemishes.
- To create different effects that can be:
  - Elegant.
  - Decorative.
  - Funky.
  - Dramatic.
  - Fun.
  - Exotic.

Make-up can make you feel more confident, but it is important that you understand how to use make-up properly. In this chapter you will start to learn about the different types of make-up product, the tools you will need to use and how to apply make-up for your clients.

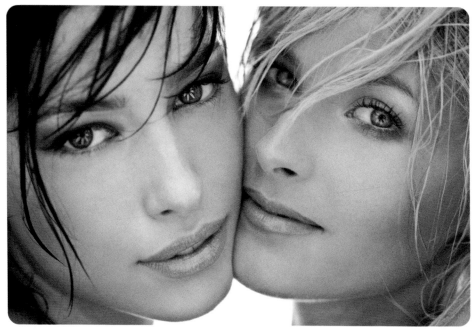

Make-up effects

Make-up can be applied immediately after a facial treatment and salons offer make-up treatments for a wide range of occasions such as:

- Weddings.
- Graduations.
- Special parties.
- Fashion shows.
- Photo shoots.

SIGNPOST FUNCTIONAL SKILLS

ICT
When you are looking at websites for information on make-up you will interact with ICT for a given purpose and you will be able to recognize and use interface features. **E3** and **L1**

For a salon to offer a wide range of make-up services the beauty therapist or make-up artist must be able to offer lots of different types of make-up, such as:

- Natural day make-up.
- Photographic make-up.
- Glamour/evening make-up.
- Camouflage make-up.

When you are carrying out a consultation with your client, you will need to consider many factors before applying any make-up:

- The occasion.
- Skin type.
- Shape of the face.
- Shape of the eyes.
- Shape of the eyebrows.
- Shape of the nose.
- Shape of the lips.
- Any skin, eye or mouth condition that may affect the make-up treatment.

The occasion

When talking and consulting with your client you will need to find out the reason why your client is having the make-up done. Where are they going? Most people think carefully about how they want to look, you will need to consider the clothes they will be wearing, the time of day or night it will be and the total image that the client wants to portray.

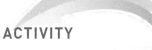

ACTIVITY

Why not find out more about different types of make-up and how it can be applied to achieve different effects. You can research information and videos from the following websites:

www.maccosmetics.co.uk
www.bobbibrowncosmetics .com

SIGNPOST PLTS

Independent enquirer

IT'S A FACT!

A person who specializes in make-up application is called a make-up artist. They can be employed to work on many exciting projects such as TV work and films, fashion shows and even photo shoots in exotic locations. It can be fun but also very hard work.

If the make-up is not planned carefully, the client may be very disappointed with the final effect.

Skin type

When applying make-up you need to consider skin type, as it will have an effect on the finished look. Make-up should be about highlighting the best features and camouflaging features the client does not like.

Shape of the face

A client's face can be improved by applying make-up correctly. It can change the shape of a face. For example, a square-shaped face will need the corner angles softening to make it appear oval. Corrective make-up can work wonders, if you know what you are doing.

You can find out more about the different types of face shapes and how to identify them in Chapter 7 'Introduction to hair care'.

Shape of the eyes

The eyes are the main focus of the face. Make-up can enhance the shape, size, colour and look of the eye area.

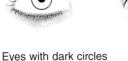

Eyes with dark circles

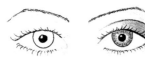

Wide set eyes

Close set eyes

 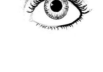

Round eyes

Prominent eyes

Overhanging lids

Deep set eyes

Downward slanting eyes

 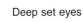

Small eyes

Narrow eyes

Oriental eyes

Shapes of the eyes

Shape of the eyebrows

Well-groomed eyebrows that are the correct shape for the face help to enhance the make-up. It is more difficult to get a good finished look if the eyebrows are too bushy and overgrown.

Shape of the nose

Many people have hang-ups about their nose – is it too big, too wide, does it have bumps or is it too long? Whatever the issue, make-up can help minimize any imperfections.

Shape of the lips

Lips come in all shapes and sizes. Make-up can achieve many different effects.

Skin, eye and mouth conditions

There are many conditions that can affect the application of make-up. Some conditions are not infectious, so the make-up application can go ahead, but others are infectious. A client with an infectious condition cannot have a make-up service carried out.

Preparing the work area for a make-up service

When preparing your work area for a make-up service for a client, you need to make sure that the environment is comfortable and that the room is ready with all the tools, materials, equipment and products you may need.

For the treatment room you will need to make sure:

- The temperature is nice and warm, but not too stuffy.
- The room is well lit.
- The music is not too loud and is in the background.

When carrying out a make-up service you will also need to make sure that the treatment room has the following specialist equipment:

- Treatment couch or make-up chair: A chair is often used for applying make-up, it is more comfortable for the client to relax in while the make-up is being applied and it makes it easier for you to apply the make-up correctly.

- Equipment trolley: To hold the equipment, tools, materials and products that you will need to use during the service.

- Beauty stool/chair: A specially designed chair/stool that you can sit on during a make-up service.

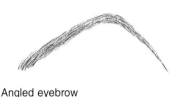

Rounded eyebrow

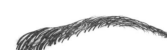

Angled eyebrow

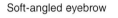

Soft-angled eyebrow

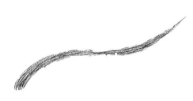

Curved eyebrow

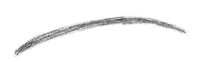

Flat eyebrow

Shapes of eyebrows

TOP TIP

Make sure you have natural light when applying day make-up, as artificial light may distort the colour and the result could be heavier than your client wanted.

When preparing your equipment, tools and materials you will need to make sure you have the following items ready in the room:

- Towels: These must be clean and soft.

- Gown/bathrobe: A clean gown is used to protect the client's modesty. Lined swing waste bin: For disposing of waste materials.

- Sterilizer: For sterilizing your tools to prevent the spread of infection.

On your equipment trolley you will need to make sure you have the following items:

Equipment/tools and materials	What they are used for
Make-up brushes 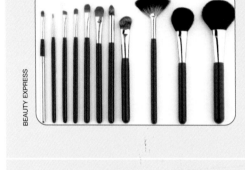	Good-quality make-up brushes are used to apply different make-up products.
Cosmetic sponges 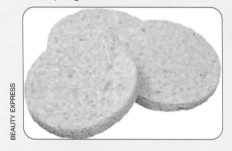	Specialized sponges for applying foundation.
Make-up palette 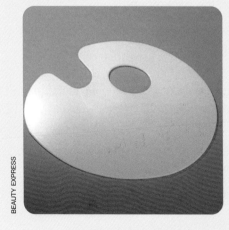	Small amounts of make-up products are placed on the palette for you to work from. This is hygienic with no risk of cross-infection.

Equipment/tools and materials	What they are used for
Disposable wands 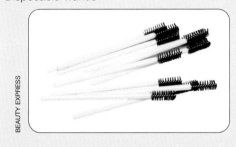	For applying mascara. They are used once only and then thrown away.
Disposable lip brushes 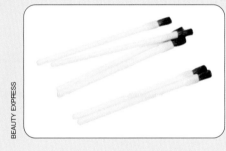	For applying lipstick. They are used once only and then thrown away.

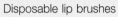

Make sure you have all the make-up products laid out on your equipment trolley before you start the treatment

HABIA AND CENGAGE LEARNING

Make-up products

Product	When and why it is used	Different types of product
Foundation	Provides the face with an even colour and texture.	● Cream ● Liquid ● Mousse

Product	When and why it is used	Different types of product
		● Gel ● Pressed powder/block
Face powder	Sets the foundation making it last all day. Helps give a smooth dry base for the rest of the make-up application.	● Pressed/block/cake ● Loose
Blusher	Adds warmth and colour to cheeks.	● Pressed powder/block ● Loose powder ● Cream ● Gel ● Liquid
Eyeshadow	Enhances and colours the eye area.	● Pressed powder/block ● Loose powder ● Cream ● Pencil/crayons ● Gel ● Water colours
Eyebrow make-up	Used to define the eyebrow.	● Pencil ● Block/powder
Eyeliner	Used to define the eye, and help make eyelashes appear longer.	● Pencil ● Liquid ● Block/cake
Mascara	Used to length, thicken and colour the eyelashes.	● Wand/liquid ● Block
Lip liner	Used to define the outer edge of the lips.	● pencil

Product	When and why it is used	Different types of product
Lipstick	Adds colour to the lips.	● Stick ● Tube ● Pot/container Pencil/crayons
Lip gloss	To add gloss and shine to the lips.	● Wand ● Tube ● Pot/container

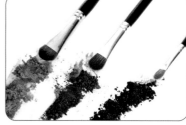

Foundation

Eye make-up and brushes

Preparing for and carrying out a basic make-up application

Like all treatments and services it is very important that good hygiene practices are followed so that the make-up is applied as safely and expertly as possible with no risk of **cross-infection**.

When carrying out a basic make-up application it is best to follow a plan. Make-up is usually applied in the following order:

1 Foundation.

2 Face powder.

3 Eyebrow pencil/colour.

4 Eyeshadow.

5 Eyepencil.

6 Eyeliner.

7 Mascara.

8 Blusher.

9 Lipliner.

10 Lipstick and gloss.

Before you start the make-up service make sure you are prepared and you have everything you need. Use hair clips to keep the client's hair secure and away from their face. Make sure the face has been properly cleansed, toned and moisturized and there is no excess grease on the skin. Blot if necessary.

Make-up application

A basic day make-up application

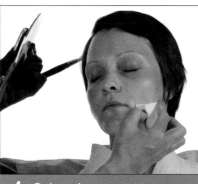

1 Select the correct type and colour of foundation; test the colour on the lower cheek area. Apply the foundation with a make-up sponge or brush to get an even finish. Apply and blend the foundation from the centre of the face outwards, taking care to blend carefully around the jaw, nose and hairline.

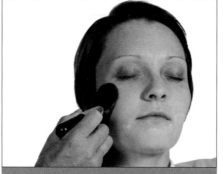

2 Select the correct colour of face powder. Apply a small amount into the palm of your hand, and with a small pad of cotton wool lightly press the powder into the skin all over the face and neck, including eyes, lids and lips. Take a large clean powder brush and remove any excess powder, finish with downward strokes. Apply extra powder under the eye area, so that it protects the skin from any excess eyeshadow that is flicked from the brush.

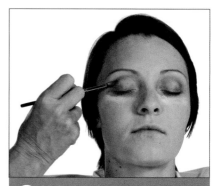

3 Using a clean eyeshadow brush, apply the eyeshadow, following the plan agreed at consultation. Start with the base shade over the entire eye area. Build the eye colour up slowly to define the eye socket and enhance the eyes.

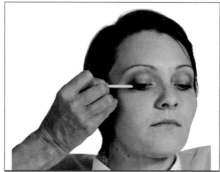

4 Using a disposable mascara wand, carefully apply two coats of mascara. First ask your client to look down, and then apply the mascara to the top of the upper lashes. Then apply to the underside of the upper lashes in an upwards direction. The lower lashes can be included if appropriate.

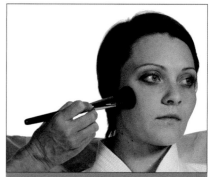

5 With a clean brush apply blusher along the cheek-bone; apply a little at a time, moving the brush outwards and upwards. Build the colour up slowly.

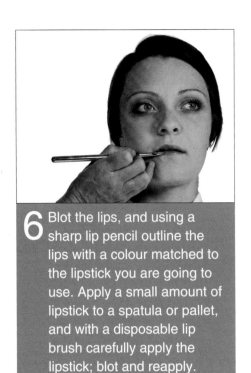

6 Blot the lips, and using a sharp lip pencil outline the lips with a colour matched to the lipstick you are going to use. Apply a small amount of lipstick to a spatula or pallet, and with a disposable lip brush carefully apply the lipstick; blot and reapply.

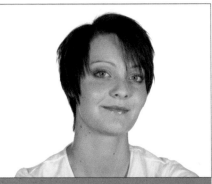

7 Remove hair clips and show the finished result to the client using a hand mirror. You can then make any final adjustments that the client wants.

TOP TIP

Apply extra face powder under the client's eye area, so that it protects the skin from excess eyeshadow that is flicked from the brush. You can then easily brush away the extra powder.

ACTIVITY

Look at the website **http://www.womanandhome.com/hair-and-beauty/makeover.html**

You can do a complete makeover on all sorts of people with different skin colour and with different ages. You can even upload you own photograph to try out different ideas for yourself.

IT'S A FACT!

You can use a concealer or corrective make-up products to disguise any blemishes or uneven skin tone such as darkness under the eyes.

SIGNPOST PLTS

Creative thinker
Independent enquirer

ICT

When you are looking and participating in activities on a website you will interact with ICT for a given purpose and you will be able to recognize and use interface features. E3 and L1

SIGNPOST FUNCTIONAL SKILLS

An evening make-up application

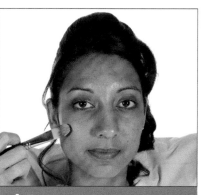

1 For an evening make-up, you can apply a foundation that is a shade darker than in the daytime, as the light is not as harsh. Apply with a make-up sponge or foundation brush to get an even finish. Apply and blend the foundation from the centre of the face outwards, taking care to blend carefully around the jaw, nose and hairline.

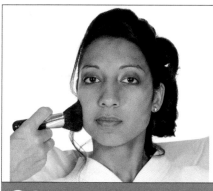

2 Select the correct colour of face powder. In the evening you can apply a powder with some shimmer or shine, as it can look very glamorous. Apply a small amount into the palm of your hand, and with a small pad of cotton wool lightly press the powder into the skin all over the face and neck, including eyes lids and lips. Take a large clean powder brush and remove any excess powder, finish with downward strokes. Apply extra face powder under the eye area so that it protects the skin from any excess eyeshadow that is flicked from the brush (but do not use shimmer powder).

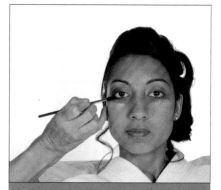

3 Using a clean eyeshadow brush, apply the eyeshadow, following the plan agreed at consultation. Start with the base shade over the entire eye area. Build the eye colour up slowly to define the eye socket and enhance the eyes. Make the eyes a strong feature, so that they are the focus of the make-up.

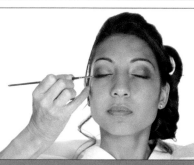

4 Apply eyeshadow carefully under the eye, just below the lower eyelash line, and blend in well. If needed apply eyeliner to the eyelash line.

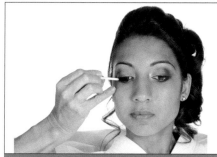

5 Using a disposable mascara wand, carefully apply two coats of mascara. First ask your client to look down, and then apply the mascara to the top of the upper lashes. Then apply to the underside of the upper lashes in an upwards direction. The lower lashes can be included if appropriate.

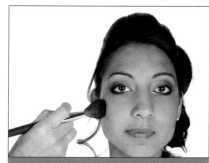

6 With a clean brush apply blusher along the cheek bone; apply a little at a time, moving the brush outwards and upwards. Build the colour up slowly. For an evening make-up you can use shimmer blusher if you client wants to be more adventurous.

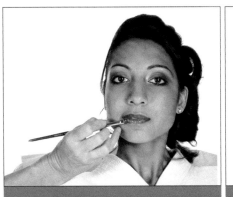

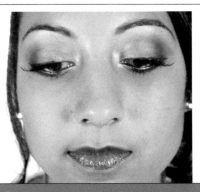

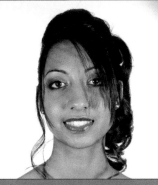

7 Blot the lips and, using a sharp lip pencil, outline the lips with a colour matched to the lipstick you are going to use. Apply a small amount of lipstick to a spatula or pallet and, with a disposable lip brush, carefully apply the lipstick. Once again you can be bolder with an evening make-up, using darker shades or a shimmer or glittery colour. When you have applied the lipstick, blot and reapply. Apply lots of gloss to bring the lips alive.

8 Show the finished result to the client using a hand mirror. Be sure to make any final adjustments that the client wants.

Finished result.

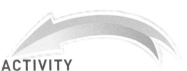

ACTIVITY

With a partner make a detailed plan or mood board for a day make-up and an evening make-up. Don't forget to include the information about factors the will affect your make-up choice, such as what the occasion is, what clothes/colours the client will be wearing and the make-up colours you will need to use.

SIGNPOST
PLTS

Teamwork
Creative thinker

English

SIGNPOST
FUNCTIONAL
SKILLS

When you complete the mood board you will:

E3 write texts with some adaptation to the intended audience

L1 write a range of texts to communicate information, ideas and opinions, using formats and styles suitable for their purpose and audience.

SIGNPOST
PLTS

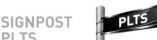

Creative thinker
Independent enquirer
Self-manager

SIGNPOST
FUNCTIONAL
SKILLS

ACTIVITY

Design a stylebook for you to use with your clients when carrying out a consultation. The book should include lots of pictures of make-up applications for different occasions. You may even want to have a page that focuses on just eyes.

ICT

When you are designing your stylebook you might look for images on the internet. If you do this you will interact with ICT for a given purpose and you will be able to recognize and use interface features. **E3** and **L1**

WHAT'S NEXT?

When you progress to Level 2 you will learn more about make-up products and what they can do. You will learn about corrective make-up techniques that you can use to change a client's look or appearance.

Face painting

Face painting is the artistic use of make-up paints that are applied to a person's face. Face painting has been used for a long time; in ancient times people camouflaged themselves with face paint to blend into their surroundings when hunting or in times of war. Today it is used more for fun, particularly with younger people when they attend parties or festivals.

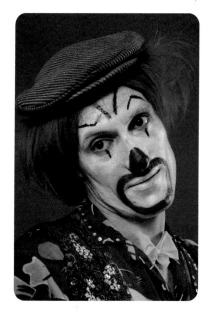

Tribal

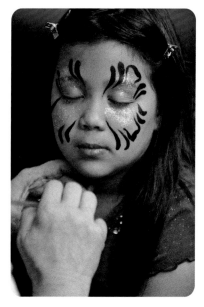

Tiger

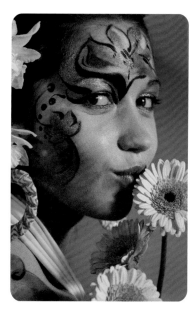

Clown

Spring

ACTIVITY

With a partner, look on the internet to see what you can find out about face painting. Can you find pictures to show how face painting has been used by different groups of people around the world? You can display the pictures you have found on a mood board and show it to your class.

SIGNPOST PLTS

Teamwork
Creative thinker
Effective participator
Independent enquirer

ICT

When you are looking at websites for information on face painting you will interact with ICT for a given purpose and you will be able to recognize and use interface features. **E3** and **L1**

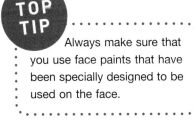

SIGNPOST
FUNCTIONAL
SKILLS

There are special water-based make-up paints that you use when face painting. If you use products that are not designed specially for a person's skin they can cause a variety of problems such as skin irritation and discomfort or severe allergic reaction.

TOP TIP

Always make sure that you use face paints that have been specially designed to be used on the face.

Face painting designs

To be a good face painter you need to be able to offer your clients a large variety of designs. Designs need to be for all age groups and for different occasions.

Face painting designs could include:

Face paint designs	Examples
Animal images	Lion, tiger, butterfly
Nature	Flowers, water, winter
Film characters	Spiderman, Batman, Cat woman
Halloween characters	Witch, skull, vampire, demons

You can get ideas from all sorts of things. Think about sport – when there is a national football match, lots of people have their national flag painted on their faces.

Before you can carry out a face painting design you need to draw the design on paper. This is called a 2D image. When you have drawn the design you can work out the different coloured paints, and the tools and materials that you will

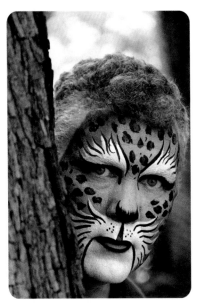

Leopard

ACTIVITY

Develop a stylebook of your different face paint designs.

For each design you will first need to plan the design on paper and then reproduce the design on to a person's face. Take pictures of the finished results so that you can show your clients.

SIGNPOST PLTS

Creative thinker
Self-manager
Independent enquirer
Reflective learner

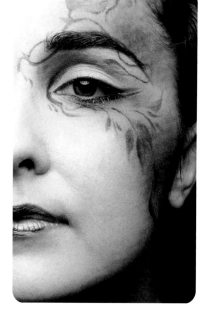

Elf face

need. You can write all this information down on your design so that you keep a record of it for future use. When you draw your design on paper don't forget that you need to transfer the design on to a client's face. When you do this it will become a 3D image.

Preparing the work area for a face painting service

When preparing the work area for a face painting service you need to make sure that the environment is comfortable and that the room is ready with all the tools, materials, equipment and products you may need.

For the room you will need to make sure:

- The temperature is nice and warm, but not too stuffy.
- The room is well lit.
- The music is not too loud and is in the background.

When carrying out a face painting service you will also need to make sure that the room has the following specialist equipment:

- Treatment couch or make-up chair: A chair is often used for applying face paints, it is more comfortable for the client to relax in while you are working.
- Equipment trolley: To hold the tools, materials and products that you will need to use during the service.
- Beauty stool/chair: A specially designed chair/stool that you can sit on while you are working.

When preparing your tools and materials, you will need to make sure you have the following items ready in the room:

- Face painting designs: A book of the designs that you can create.
- Towels: These must be clean and soft.
- Headband: To protect and secure the client's hair out of the way while you are working.
- Gown/bathrobe: A clean gown is used to protect the client's own clothes. Lined swing waste bin: For disposing of waste materials.
- Sterilizer: For sterilizing your tools, to prevent the spread of infection.

On your equipment trolley you will need to make sure you have the following items:

- Good-quality art brushes of different sizes and shapes to enable you to cover large areas, create bold strokes, draw thin lines or paint dots.
- Brush holder or container to hold all your brushes.
- Specialized sponges for applying face paints and blending.
- Container for your sponges.
- Containers for clean water.

- Tissues or baby wipes for wiping your hands.
- A hand mirror.
- Face paint products.
- Face glitters.
- Face transfers.

Consulting with your client

Remember that before you carry out a face painting service you need to carry out a consultation with your client to find out exactly what kind of design your client wants.

It can be very useful to have a portfolio or file of your designs so that you can show your client the types of design that you can create.

You will also need to check that the client has no skin conditions that may stop you carrying out the service. Look out for the following signs:

- Redness.
- Open sores.
- Cuts and abrasions.

If you are unsure about checking for skin conditions you will need to get support from a more experienced team member.

You then need to agree the face paint design and any adjustments to the design before you start.

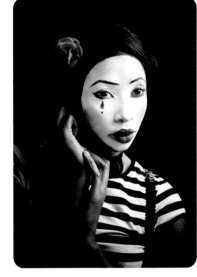

Mime face

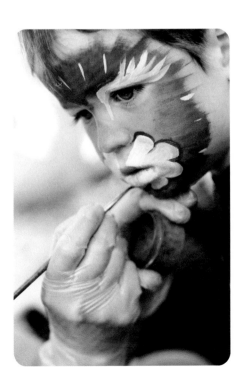

Face being painted

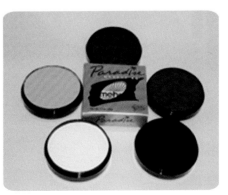

Aqua colours used for face painting

Carrying out a face painting design

A simple facemask

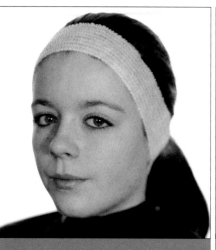

1 Make sure that your client's clothes are well protected and the hair is kept off the face.

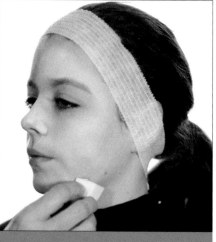

2 Use white face paint as the base and apply evenly with a sponge on to the whole face.

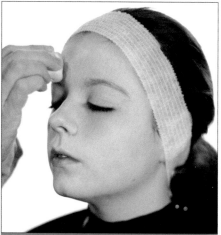

3 Use a second colour to create a mask shape that covers the eye area and across the nose.

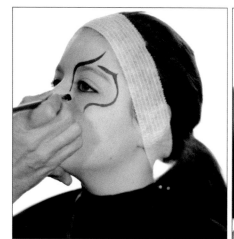

4 With a steady hand draw outline shapes around the edges of the mask to give the mask definition. The outline can be of any design but it is better to use a dark colour face paint such as black.

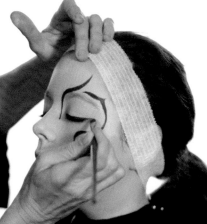

5 Using a very fine brush and your black paint draw a black line on the top eyelid close to the eyelashes.

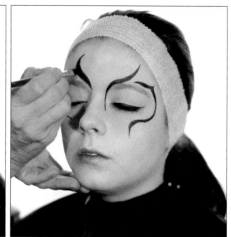

6 Repeat the design on the other side of the face. The design can be slightly different or it can be exactly the same.

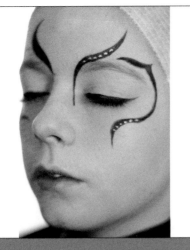

7 Apply small dots on to the black outline design. You can use different colours, but make sure you pick colours that will stand out from the black paint; we have used white face paint.

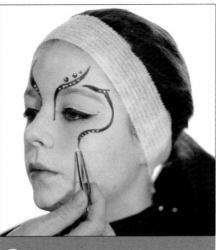

8 Complete the design by using self-adhesive jewels to add sparkle. You can apply the jewels with your fingers or with tweezers. Tweezers make it easier to adjust the jewels into the correct position.

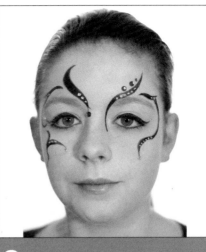

9 Finished result.

A tiger

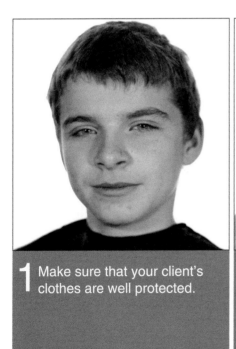

1 Make sure that your client's clothes are well protected.

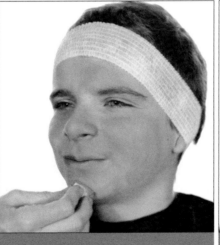

2 Apply a base coat of orange face paint evenly over the face using a make-up sponge. Make sure the lips are covered.

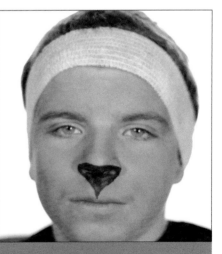

3 Using black paint draw an outline of a triangle across the tip of the nose down to a point at the centre of the upper lip. Colour in the triangle.

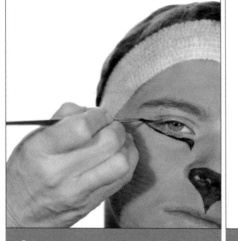

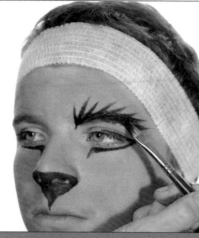

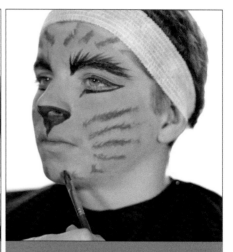

4 Use the black paint and a fine brush to outline the eye. The eye needs to appear wider and longer. Start under the eye near the nose and draw a line to the outer corner of the eye. Then apply the paint in a thin line along the eyelid close to the eyelashes.

5 Colour the eyebrows using black paint to create strong, bold eyebrows. Use a brush to create a feathering effect.

6 Along the cheeks and outer edges of the face draw feather-like/zigzag lines to create the impression of fur. Use both black and white paint to create the fur.

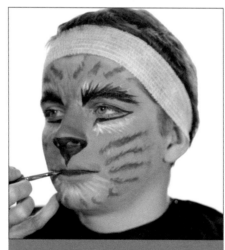

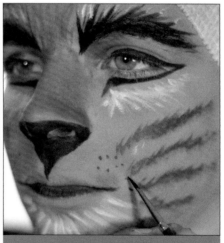

7 Mix a little black paint to the orange base paint or just use a darker shade of the base paint to colour in the nose area. As you work from the tip of the nose towards the top of the nose between the eyes, start to fan out the colour so that it blends into the original base colour and also looks like fur. Then use black paint to create a fine line across the lips. Extend the lip past the lips to make it appear longer.

8 Apply black dots and thin lines to the outer corners of the mouth up towards the cheek area to create the whiskers.

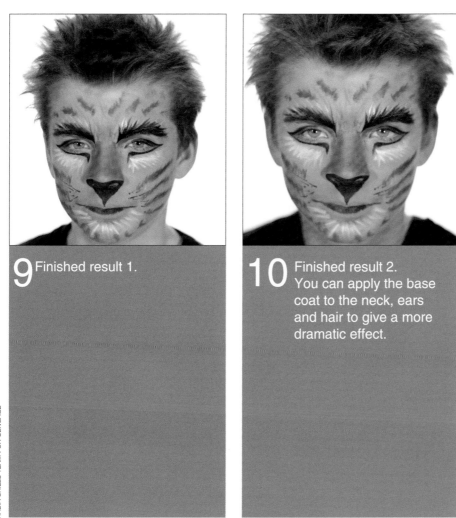

HABIA SKILLS TEAM FOR CENGAGE

9 Finished result 1.

10 Finished result 2.
You can apply the base coat to the neck, ears and hair to give a more dramatic effect.

Removal of make-up products

Removing face paints is very simple; because they are water-based paints, they are easy to remove with water. For the best results use mild soap and water.

What you have learnt

- The importance of good skincare:
  - How skin can be affected by diet and the environment.
- The basic structure and function of the skin:
  - Understanding the different layers of the skin.
  - How skin protects us.
  - The different skin types.

○ An awareness of different skin conditions that may affect a treatment or service.

● The bone structure:

○ An awareness of the different bones of the head and face.

● Preparing the work area:

○ How to prepare the treatment room.

○ The different types of equipment, tools, materials and products that are needed to carry out facial and make-up services.

● How to carrying out a basic skincare treatment:

○ The step-by-step procedure for carrying out a basic facial treatment.

● How to carrying out basic make-up applications:

○ The step-by-step procedure of a basic day make-up.

○ The step-by-step procedure of a basic evening make-up.

○ The step-by-step procedure for carrying out a face painting design.

○ How to remove face paints.

ASSESSMENT ACTIVITIES

Activity 1 E 3 and L1

These are multiple choice questions. Read through each question carefully. When you have finished, tick the correct answer.

1   The number of layers that make up the skin:

   a. 1   c. 5
   b. 3   d. 7.

2   The top layer of the skin is called:

   a. Dermis.
   b. Subcutaneous layer.
   c. Cuticle.
   d. Epidermis.

3   The number of bones in the skull:

   a. 14   c. 22
   b. 18   d. 24

4   How many main skin types are there?

   a. 3
   b. 4
   c. 5
   d. 6

5   What type of skin condition has an animal living on or in our body?

   a. Viral condition.   c. Parasitic condition.
   b. Bacterial condition.   d. Fungal condition.

6   What is the main purpose of a moisturizer?

   a. To clean the skin.
   b. To prevent the skin taking in moisture.
   c. To refresh the skin.
   d. To prevent the skin getting to dry.

7   In what order is a basic facial treatment carried out when you are not using a facial scrub or mask?

   a. Cleanse, tone and moisturize.
   b. Tone, cleanse and moisturize.
   c. Moisturize, tone and cleanse.
   d. Cleanse, moisturize and tone.

8   What is the main purpose of a foundation make-up product?

   a. To protect the skin.
   b. To give even skin colour.
   c. To give warmth to the cheek area.
   d. To define the face shape.

9 Which make-up product is used to define the edge of the eye?

a. Eyeliner.
b. Eyebrow pencil.
c. Eyeshadow.
d. Mascara.

10 What is the main purpose of a blusher?

a. To give colour to the eyes.
b. To highlight the brow bone.
c. To highlight the cheek bone.
d. To give colour to the jaw line.

Activity 2 E3 and L1

Work with a partner or split into two teams. Choose a letter and answer the question. When you have answered the question correctly, mark off the square. See who can correctly answer the questions to complete a straight line across the grid. You can block the way of your partner or other team to stop them winning!

C	E	L	A
M	B	F	E
S	T	O	S
N	A	B	C

Letter	Question
C	Which C describes looking after your skin?
M	Which M describes the natural colour pigment of skin?
E	Which E is the top layer of the skin?
S	Which S the third layer of the skin?
E	Which E describes a function of the skin?
S	Which S is a natural oil found on the skin?
S	Which S is the term used for the group of bones to the head and face?
L	Which L is the only bone that can move?
S	Which S describes exactly similar items on each side or facing each other?
M	Which M is long lasting and can heal itself?
O	Which O is a skin type?
C	Which C is a skin type?
B	Which B is a type of skin condition?
S	Which S is used to apply make-up?
C	Which C is used to cleanse the skin?
T	Which T is used in a facial treatment?
S	Which S is used to remove dead skin cells?

Letter	Question
A	Which A is used in a cleanser?
E	Which E enables us to see?
L	Which L is used to colour the lips?
A	Which A is used in a toner?
T	Which T is the name given to beauty services?
B	Which B is used to give colour to the cheeks?
F	Which F is used as a make-up base?
L	Which L is used around the eyes?
A	Which A is used to describe a person who applies make-up?
A	Which A is a function of the skin?
F	Which F describes the front part of the skull?
L	Which L describes the different levels of the skin?
C	Which C is another name for the bones of the head?
M	Which M is the name given to face products?
C	Which C is used to find out what treatment your client wants done?
F	Which F is the term used for a skincare treatment?
N	Which N is a skin type?
N	Which N is used to describe a soft day make-up look?

5
The art of photographic make-up

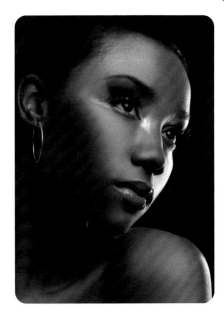

"The best thing is to look natural, but it takes make-up to look natural.

CALVIN KLEIN, AMERICAN FASHION DESIGNER, B.1942

In this chapter you are going to learn about:

- The importance of the preparation procedures for photographic make-up.

- The safe and hygienic procedures that must be followed.

- How to select and use products, tools and equipment for photographic make-up application.

- The factors that affect photographic make-up application.

- The sequence in which make-up products should be applied.

- Providing aftercare advice.

- How to evaluate the effectiveness of the make-up application.

- The work of a photographic make-up artist.

Introduction

Becoming a photographic make-up artist is just one of the many career pathways you can choose when you have completed a qualification in beauty therapy. This is a very exciting, fashion-related area to work in. Many photographic make-up artists specialize in make-up for special occasions such as bridal parties or evening events. It can also be very high profile. Some make-up artists also work in television on photo shoots and preparing models for catwalk shows. One day, the results of your work could be on the front cover of the most exclusive glossy magazines. Applying the make-up for photographic work is not that different to an everyday make-up application. But the colours you choose and the products you use must be carefully selected and applied. Your make-up application must meet the requirements of your client – who may not be the model you are working on. You may also have to work with a team of other people. Some people may be dressing your model, others doing the hair. Read this chapter and see how you can use your most creative skills.

The importance of the preparation procedures for photographic make-up

In Chapter 4, 'Skincare, make-up and face painting', you can read about the preparations you must make for a make-up application. Preparation for photographic make-up is slightly different. Some clients may come to you in the salon. You may get a bride and her attendants as well as the bride's mother in for a make-up session. Sometimes, the bride wants to get ready in her own home, so you may have to travel. For some work, you may have to apply the make-up in a photographer's studio, backstage at a catwalk or fashion show, in small cramped changing rooms or in large airy dressing rooms. So, you have to be prepared for anything! You may even have to work outside.

Make-up kit and storage

You must have your kit of products and equipment ready for the make-up application. In Chapter 4 you can find details of all the products and equipment you are likely to need. If you are working in the salon, you will have everything to hand. But if you have to travel you will need to have a storage box to keep your products, tools and equipment in. The box will also be required to transport your kit to your location. The box should have a lid to protect your products, tools and equipment. It should be light, but tough and easy to carry.

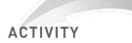

ACTIVITY

Use the internet to find a storage box that would be light, tough and easy to take with you if you are asked to carry out a photographic make-up application at a location outside the salon. When you have investigated the storage options for transporting make-up, write a brief report about the options that are available.

SIGNPOST
FUNCTIONAL
SKILL

ICT
Use the internet to investigate the storage solutions for transporting make-up to various locations. When you do this, you will:
E3 use simple searches to find web-based sources of information
L1 use search techniques to locate and select relevant information.

SIGNPOST
FUNCTIONAL
SKILL

English and ICT
When you write your report about the different types of make-up storage boxes, you could use a word processing package for the text and to insert images of storage boxes that you find. When you do this, you will:
E3 plan, draft and organize writing; sequence writing logically and clearly
L1 present information in a logical sequence; write clearly and coherently, including an appropriate level of detail
E3 enter, edit and format information including text
L1 apply editing, formatting and layout to meet needs, including text.

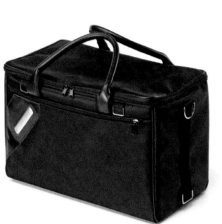

© AMABILIA PROFESSIONAL CASES

Storage boxes for photographic make-up must be easy to transport

Preparing for the photographic make-up application

When preparing for a photographic make-up you need to know who you are working for, what the end result will be and where you are going to be working.

The client

If you are doing photographic make-up for a bride or on someone for another special occasion, the client will be the person you are working on.

But sometimes you will be working on a model who is not your 'client'. The person who has the make-up application will not be the person to tell you how they want to look. Your 'client' may be the photographer, the organizer of the catwalk show or even the fashion editor of a glossy magazine. They may tell you exactly what is required or they may ask you to come to the photo shoot with some ideas. If you are asked to come prepared with ideas you may want to make a mood board to show others the results you want to achieve. You can read about how to make a mood board in Chapter 3, 'Understanding and using colour'.

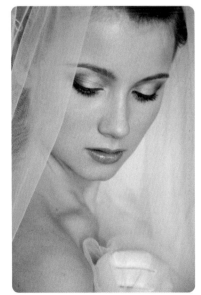

Your client may be a bride

The model

Whether the model is a regular client or one who is new to you, you must still carry out a consultation as you would for any make-up application. In particular, you must check for any **contra-indications** and skin sensitivity.

This is particularly important if you are going to apply special effect products such as cosmetic glitters or jewellery that may be applied to the skin. Check that your model is not allergic to latex products that may be found in the glue used for false lash application.

IT'S A FACT!

A contra-indication is a condition the client may have that will prevent you from carrying out treatment or service. For example, an infectious disease of the skin would be a contra-indication.

Final result

As well as how the final result will look, you will need to find out how it will be seen. Will the final result be seen very close up, or from a distance? In daylight or under artificial lights? Which lighting conditions will be used for the photograph? It may be low, moody lighting, or very bright spotlights. Some lighting may be coloured, which will affect the colours that you use for the make-up. The photographs could be taken during daylight or in the evening as the natural light is fading.

Working space

You need to ensure that you have a clear working space and good lighting for the application of the make-up. This will not be a problem if you are working in the salon. If you are working in a photographic studio, you may be able to work near to the lights where the photographs are taken. Some make-up storage boxes have built-in lights. But do remember that, depending on your location, you may not have electricity to connect to.

Products

You must be prepared with all the products you are going to need for your make-up application. If you are doing the make-up for a special occasion, you will probably have a **trial run**, so you will know exactly what products are required.

For other types of photographic make-up, you may have been given a **brief**, or attended a planning meeting before the day of the photo shoot. Then you can plan which products you are going to need.

You need to find out if you have to provide additional products and accessories over and above that which you normally have in your kit. For example, you may be asked to provide a particular style of false eyelashes, cosmetic glitters or jewellery for the skin. You may also have to style the hair to complement your make-up, so you may need some basic hairdressing equipment.

IT'S A FACT!

A brief is a description of the photographic project you will be working on and an outline of the work you are required to complete.

Kit and equipment for a photographic make-up artist

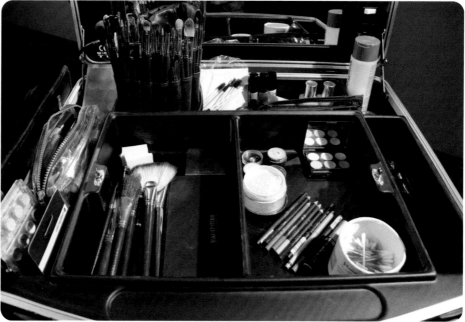

The safe and hygienic procedures that must be followed

If you are completing your make-up in your salon, you will be able to control the environment you are working in. But, if you are working outside the salon, you must still make sure that your area is a safe and hygienic place to work in:

- You could be working where there are lots of loose cables, so you need to be careful that both you and your models are aware of where the cables are to avoid tripping and falling.

- You must ensure that the same rules for sterilization apply when you are on location as when you are working in a salon.

- You will not be able to easily transport liquids, so use sanitizing hand cleaners or individual antiseptic wipes to cleanse your hands before you work on every model.

- While working, brushes and other tools can be sterilized with quick-drying brush cleaner. They must be washed thoroughly at the end of every session with anti-bacterial soap or shampoo.

- You must never '**double dip**' tools into make-up. Remove make-up using a sterilized spatula and apply make-up with single use applicators for eyeliner, mascara, lipstick etc. Throw away the single use applicators after each application.

- If your model has a skin condition that is normally a contra-indication but the make-up must still be applied, wear disposable gloves to avoid cross-infection. For example, a bride may have a cold sore on her mouth or an infected spot, but she will still want to look nice for her wedding.

- Gowns and towels must be freshly laundered for each model.

WEB LINK

This website has lots of information that is useful for a professional photographic make-up artist, including top tips for hygienic working practices: http://www.thepromake-upshop.com/

TOP TIP   If a client shows an **allergic reaction** to any of the products you have used, you must remove the product immediately and, if necessary, tell your model to seek medical advice.

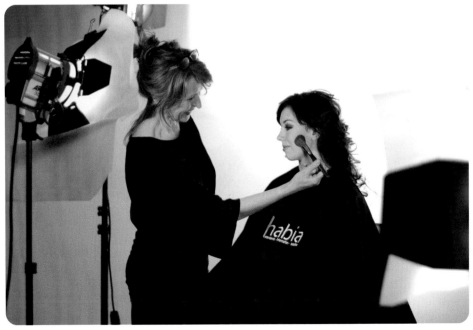

Photographic make-up artist working at a photo shoot

WWW

WEB LINK

The Portable Appliance Test (PAT) is a legal requirement to ensure that electrical equipment is safe to use. If retailed equipment is found to be unsafe, it is recalled. Check out this website of recalled equipment. It contains hair dryers and hair straighteners that you might take with you to a photo shoot. http://www.pat-testing.info/recallnotice/index.htm

- Ensure your model is seated at a suitable height so that you avoid excessive bending and stress on your own body.

- Tie your hair back so that you are not constantly pushing it away from your face.

- Any electrical equipment you use must be safe. Portable electrical equipment must be checked by a qualified person and have a portable appliance test (PAT) certificate to ensure it is safe to use.

How to select and use products, tools and equipment for photographic make-up application

You can read about the products, tools and equipment required for a make-up application in Chapter 4, 'Skincare, make-up and face painting'. Make-up brushes need to be chosen very carefully for photographic make-up to ensure the flawless results that will be expected and may be seen very close up.

Products

You can read all about the types of cleansing, toning, moisturizing and make-up product you may need in Chapter 4. You must ensure that you have wide range of different types of product for all skin conditions. You will also need a wide range of colours of all the different types of make-up. If you are not working on a regular client, you may not know what you are going to need for your model until you arrive at your location.

You will need to have a range of both matt and shimmery eye colours in every colour you can imagine. Nude and natural colours will be required for everyday looks, as well as colours for creating **'smoky' eyes** and high fashion/avant garde looks. Concealers, foundations, blushers and highlighters are required for the full range of racial skin tones.

Professional make-up ranges have lots of colours for every type of client

TOP TIP
You may have to carry out a make-up with a historic theme, so it is very useful to research the make-up trends of ancient and modern history.

TOP TIP
Professional make-up artists can use a specially designed colour wheel to predict the end results of colour mixing.

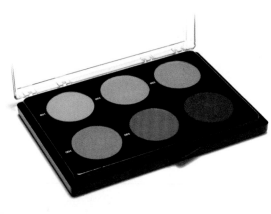

SCREENFACE FOUNDATION PALETTE

It is possible to make your own colours of make-up by mixing products on your palette. For example, you can mix different shades of lipstick to achieve the exact shade required. You can mix moisturizer with the foundation for a lighter cover or mix different shades together to get a perfect match for the skin tone. Read more about mixing colour in Chapter 3, 'Understanding and using colour'.

Colour wheel for make-up artists

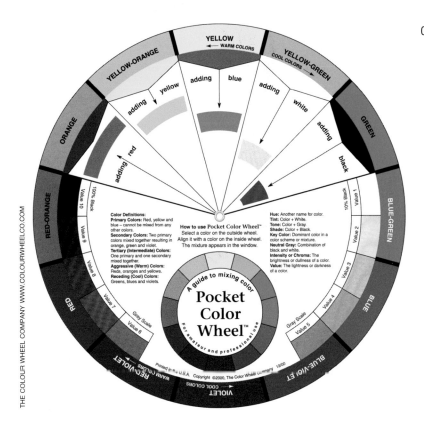

THE COLOUR WHEEL COMPANY WWW.COLOURWHEELCO.COM

Tools

You need to be prepared for a photo shoot with a wide range of cosmetic brushes.

Brush	Purpose	Tip
Concealer brush	To apply concealer to dark circles around the eye or to spots or blemishes.	The bristles must not be too hard as they could damage the delicate areas around the eye.
Foundation brush	For the application of liquid and cream foundations.	Use a flat, tapered brush to get close to the narrow areas around the nose and mouth.

WWW.LOUISEYOUNGCOSMETICS.COM

Brush	Purpose	Tip
Powder brush 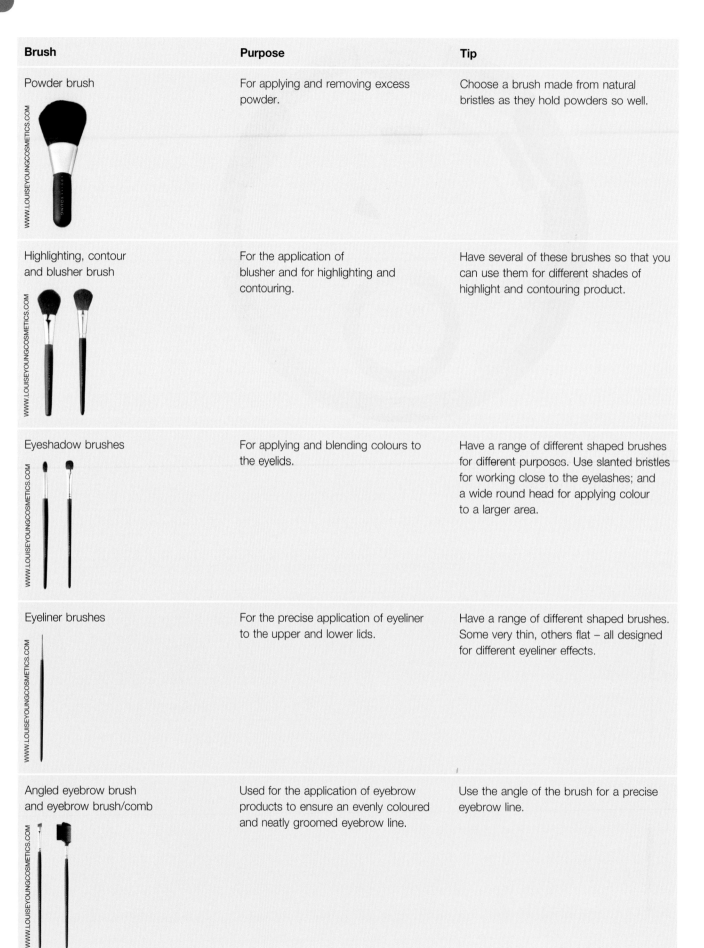 WWW.LOUISEYOUNGCOSMETICS.COM	For applying and removing excess powder.	Choose a brush made from natural bristles as they hold powders so well.
Highlighting, contour and blusher brush WWW.LOUISEYOUNGCOSMETICS.COM	For the application of blusher and for highlighting and contouring.	Have several of these brushes so that you can use them for different shades of highlight and contouring product.
Eyeshadow brushes WWW.LOUISEYOUNGCOSMETICS.COM	For applying and blending colours to the eyelids.	Have a range of different shaped brushes for different purposes. Use slanted bristles for working close to the eyelashes; and a wide round head for applying colour to a larger area.
Eyeliner brushes WWW.LOUISEYOUNGCOSMETICS.COM	For the precise application of eyeliner to the upper and lower lids.	Have a range of different shaped brushes. Some very thin, others flat – all designed for different eyeliner effects.
Angled eyebrow brush and eyebrow brush/comb WWW.LOUISEYOUNGCOSMETICS.COM	Used for the application of eyebrow products to ensure an evenly coloured and neatly groomed eyebrow line.	Use the angle of the brush for a precise eyebrow line.

Brush	Purpose	Tip
Lip brush 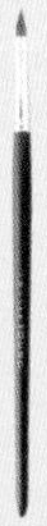	For the application of lipstick and for blending lip liner.	Use the brush to mix your own shades of lipstick on your make-up palette.
Disposable tools: 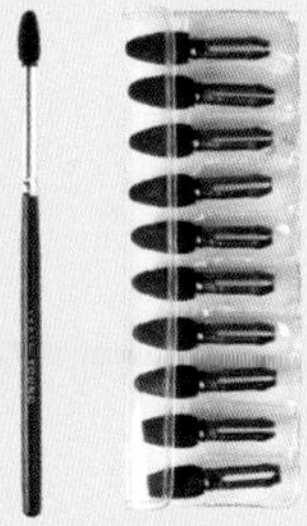	For the application of make-up to the face, eyes and lips.	Throw away after use.

- Mascara wands
- Eyeshadow applicators
- Lip brushes
- Eyeliner brushes
- Highlight and contour brushes
- Make-up sponges

WWW.LOUISEYOUNGCOSMETICS.COM

Equipment

Item	Purpose	Tip
Gown 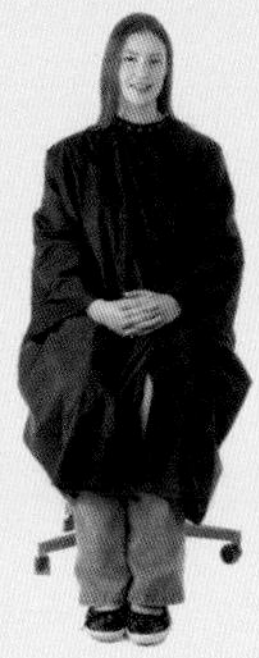	To protect model's clothing during the make-up application.	Ensure the gown and towel are freshly laundered for each new model.

COURTESY OF MAJESTIC TOWELS LTD (COPYRIGHT HOLDER)

Item	Purpose	Tip
Tweezers IMAGE BY SORISA	To tidy eyebrows.	Sterilize before use with a sterile wipe. Have a range of different tips.
Eyelash curlers 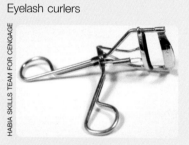 HABIA SKILLS TEAM FOR CENGAGE	To curl the eyelashes.	Sterilize before use with a sterile wipe.
Portable make-up chair 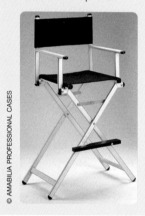 © AMABILIA PROFESSIONAL CASES	To ensure the comfort of both model and make-up artist.	Ensure it is light enough to carry. Some chairs have useful side tables. Others have covers for transportation.
Colour wheel THE COLOUR WHEEL COMPANY. WWW.COLORWHEELCO.COM	Use as a reminder of the primary and secondary colours of pigment.	Move the colour wheel around to confirm the results of colours you want to mix.

WHAT'S NEXT?

You can progress from a Level 1 qualification in hair and beauty to a NVQ Level 2 beauty therapy qualification following a make-up route. You can progress from there to NVQ Level 3 beauty therapy make-up. When you do this, you complete a unit for designing and creating fashion and photographic make-up.

Item	Purpose	Tip
Hand-held mirror IMAGE BY ELLISONS	To show the finished result to your model.	Buy one that fits easily into your storage box.
Brush holders IMAGE BY ELLISONS	To keep clean, sterile brushes off surfaces.	Collapsible containers will take up less space in your kit box.
Waste container IMAGE BY ELLISONS	For collecting single use applicators for disposal.	Collapsible containers will take up less space in your storage box.
Pencil sharpener HABIA SKILLS TEAM FOR CENGAGE	For ensuring a sterile application of lip and eyeliner.	Have a sealed unit to contain sharpening waste. Sterilize after use.
False eyelashes HABIA SKILLS TEAM FOR CENGAGE	For lengthening and increasing the density of natural lashes.	Have a range of different types, strip and individual.

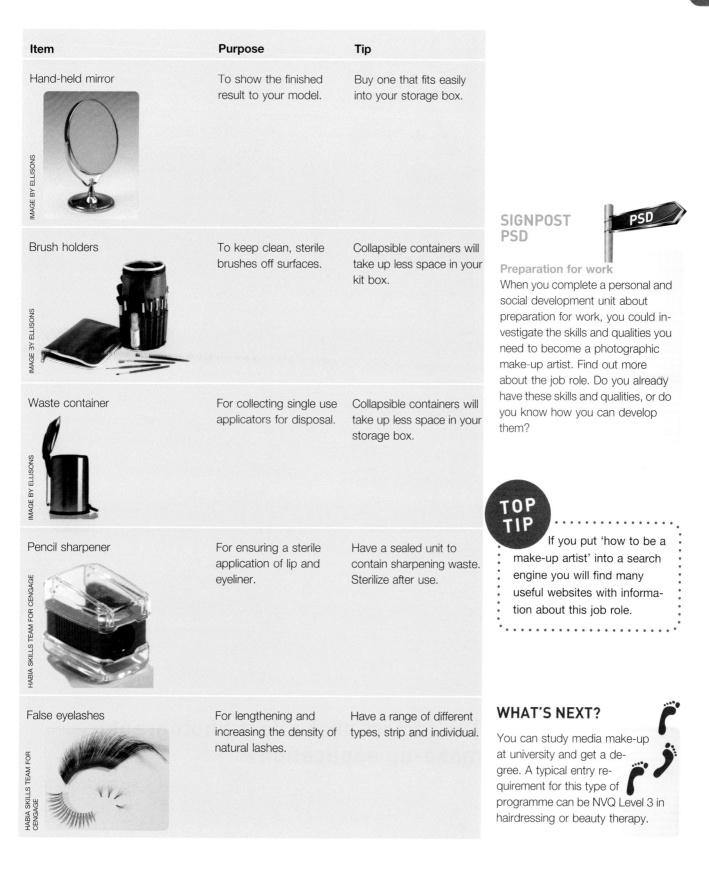

SIGNPOST PSD

Preparation for work

When you complete a personal and social development unit about preparation for work, you could investigate the skills and qualities you need to become a photographic make-up artist. Find out more about the job role. Do you already have these skills and qualities, or do you know how you can develop them?

TOP TIP

If you put 'how to be a make-up artist' into a search engine you will find many useful websites with information about this job role.

WHAT'S NEXT?

You can study media make-up at university and get a degree. A typical entry requirement for this type of programme can be NVQ Level 3 in hairdressing or beauty therapy.

ACTIVITY

Picture yourself setting up a new business as a self-employed photographic make-up artist. You need to invest in a range of products, tools and equipment. Make a list of everything you may need. Then carry out some research to calculate the total costs of buying your start-up kit. You could look on the internet for suppliers of beauty products, or visit your local beauty wholesale showrooms.

Item	Purpose	Tip
Make-up palette	For mixing and blending make-up before use.	Choose a palette with individual mixing wells to contain products.
Spatulas	For transferring make-up products.	Use single use spatulas and throw away; or use stainless steel which can be sterilized.

SIGNPOST FUNCTIONAL SKILL

ICT

Use the internet to investigate the tools, products and equipment you need to buy to be a self-employed photographic make-up artist. When you do this, you will:

E3 use simple searches to find web-based sources of information

L1 use search techniques to locate and select relevant information.

SIGNPOST FUNCTIONAL SKILL

Mathematics

Calculate the total costs to buy the tools, products and equipment for a self-employed photographic make-up artist. When you do this, you will:

E3 apply mathematics to obtain answers to simple given practical problems by completing simple calculations involving money

L1 apply mathematics in an organized way to find solutions to straightforward, practical problems and to solve problems requiring calculations including money.

SIGNPOST PLTS

Independent enquirer
Creative thinker

The factors that affect photographic make-up application

There are some factors that may affect the application of photographic make-up. You need to consider the following before you begin:

- Purpose.
- Light.
- Colour.
- Time.
- Finished result.

Purpose

The purpose for a photographic make-up will be discussed at planning meetings. A planning meeting may be between you and your client, such as for wedding or special occasion make-up. Or you may be at a meeting with many other people who will also be involved in the event. Make sure you pay close attention to what is required. Takes notes or draw sketches to remind you – it may be some time between the planning meeting and the event.

Light

Light can affect the application of the photographic make-up and the finished result. You need to make sure that you have sufficient light to apply the make-up so that you can check for any flaws that may show up under the lights used by the photographer. Most photographers will take some test shots and you may have to adjust the make-up you have applied. The photographer will use lighting to create different effects. Direct light may show up flaws in the skin or the make-up, but can be very dramatic. The photographer can also redirect harsh light by using a special photography umbrella which will soften the light on the model's face. Light will also reflect off the make-up used. Sometimes a matt result is required, at other times, light reflecting products are used to emphasize cheek and eyebrow bones.

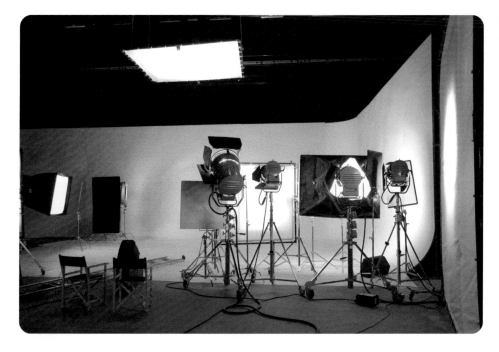

Photographers will use different lighting effects

Colour

Which colours are you going to use on your model? You may be able to decide this, or you may be told what to use. Your client may want a very natural look, so nude and natural colours can be used to create an almost 'no make-up' look. Sometimes, you may have to adapt the model's make-up so that you go from a day to an evening look. You can do this by adding a more dramatic eyeline and using darker, more intense colours on the eyes and lips. You may be asked to use colours that are related to the theme of the photo shoot. For example, you may be asked to represent the seasonal colours of autumn by using warm reds

ACTIVITY

This activity can be carried out by everyone in your class. Split into small teams and investigate the typical make-up trends for different periods of time in ancient and recent history. Each team should investigate a different era. Make up a mood board to show the fashions, hairstyles and colours that were used for your chosen era. Then carry out a makeover for your chosen era on a model. Photograph the results of your make-up and display the images along with your mood boards. Evaluate your work. Write a short report about what you did well. Plan how you would improve something if you repeated the activity.

SIGNPOST PLTS

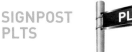

Teamworker
Creative thinker
Effective participator
Self-manager
Reflective learner
Independent enquirer

SIGNPOST PSD

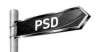

Working as part of a group
When you have completed your class activity to investigate the styles of make-up of an historical era, you will know how to work with others in appropriate ways. You will be able to set ground rules of teamwork and agree the tasks that you each carry out. You will also be able to review the work of your team members.

and coppers, or for a winter theme, the ice cold colours of blue and grey. Or the colours may be used to complement those of the client or model's clothing. Colours may be used to represent a period of history. For example the white faces of the Elizabethan period, the powdered faces of men and women in the eighteenth century. Or, more recent history, the dark, lined eyes of the 1960s and the bright eye colours of the 1970s.

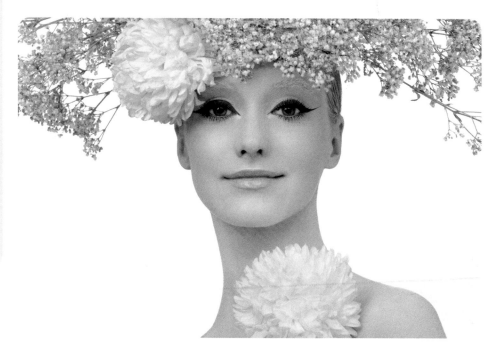

A model has make-up to reflect the theme of winter colours

A model has make-up to reflect the fashions of the 1960s

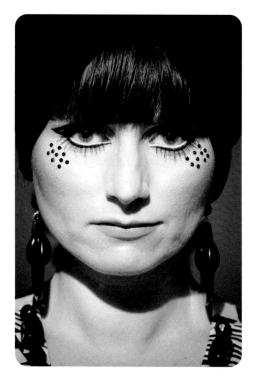

Time

How to plan your own time is a very important skill for a photographic make-up artist. First, you need to find out how much time you have to complete your make-up. Will you be the only make-up artist, or will you be working in a team with others? If you are on your own, you may have a number of models to complete. You need to find out which model must be completed first. You must ensure that you work to the times you are allocated. Falling behind could mean that others cannot complete their work on time. This could be very costly for the photo shoot.

Finished result

Will the final result be photographed in black and white, or in colour? For black and white photography, the colour of the make-up is less important than the shade. The shade you use should be stronger than that for colour photography. For example, red and purple colours always look darker in a black and white image, while pinks and yellow will look lighter.

The sequence in which make-up products should be applied

Bridal make-up (colour)

ACTIVITY

Make a plan for completing the make-up for a wedding party. You will be the only make-up artist. You have to make up the bride, one bridesmaid, one flower girl and the bride's mum. The wedding takes place at 2.00 pm. What time will you need to start? How long will you allow for each person? What time will you need to finish? Remember the bride will need time to dress in her wedding outfit.

SIGNPOST
PLTS

Independent enquirer

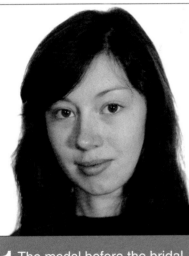

1 The model before the bridal make-up application.

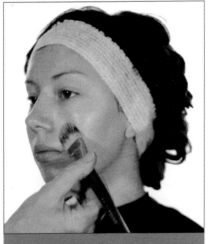

2 Following cleansing, toning and moisturising, the foundation was colour matched to the skin tone by applying some to the jaw line. The foundation was evenly applied using a flat, bristle foundation brush and a make-up sponge to remove excess foundation. The application began at the centre of the face and was blended out towards the jaw and hair line.

TOP TIP

Lower the chin so that any shadows on the face can be seen. Use a lighter concealer for dark areas and the same colour as the foundation for skin imperfections.

TOP TIP

When applying cream blusher, use a brush made from synthetic fibres

TOP TIP

Use the handle of the eyebrow brush to calculate where the start and end of the brow line should be.

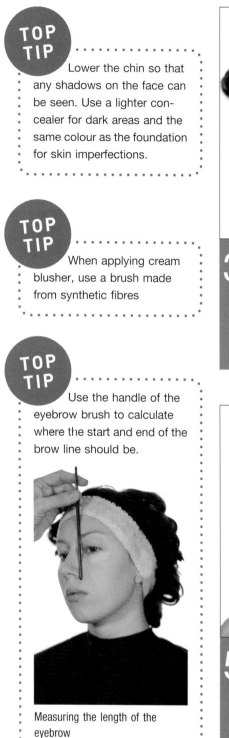

Measuring the length of the eyebrow

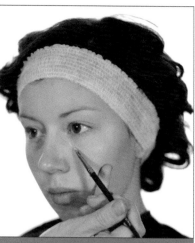

3 Concealer was applied to remove dark circles and skin imperfections. The concealer was applied with a brush and blended with a cotton bud.

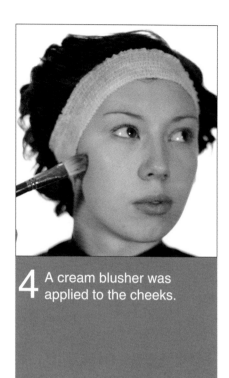

4 A cream blusher was applied to the cheeks.

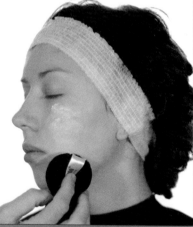

5 Powder was applied over the face and eyelids using a clean powder puff in a rolling action. Excess powder was removed using a large powder brush.

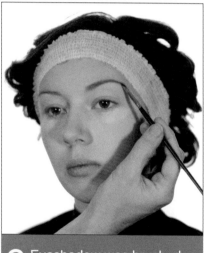

6 Eyeshadow was brushed onto the eyebrows using an angled eyebrow brush to create a natural line.

TOP TIP

Leave a layer of powder under the eye to catch eyeshadow colours that fall onto the face.

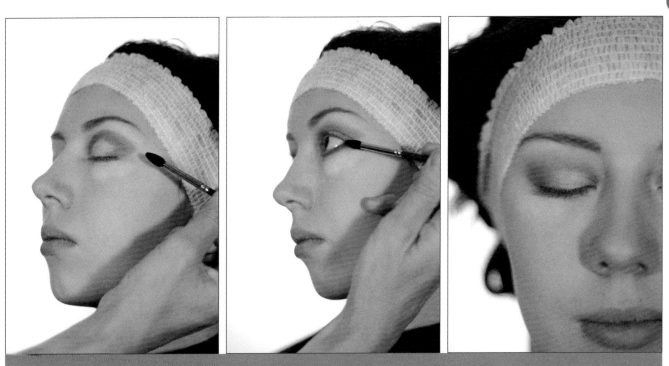

7 A cream-coloured, matt eyeshadow was applied to the whole of the eyelid from the lash to the brow line to provide a base for other colours. Brown eyeshadow was applied to the socket line and blended using a cotton bud. The same colour was applied under the eye using the tip of the eyeshadow applicator for a stronger effect. A shimmery gold eyeshadow was applied to the inside corner of the upper and lower lid.

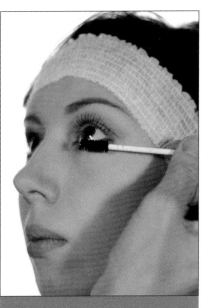

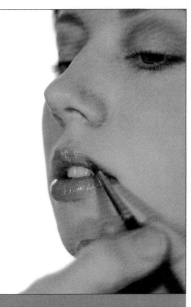

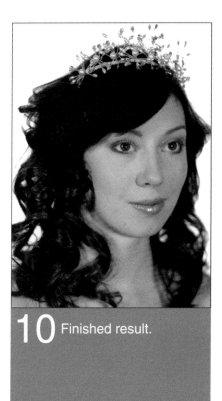

8 Mascara was applied using a disposable mascara wand, first on the top of the upper lashes and then to the underneath. Once dry, mascara was applied to the lower lashes.

9 A neutral-toned lip gloss was applied with a lip brush.

10 Finished result.

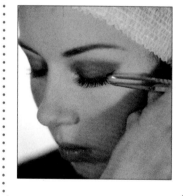

Photographic make-up (colour)

The photographic make-up was applied as steps 1–5 bridal make-up.

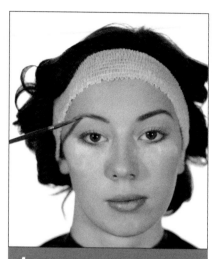

1 To define the eyebrows they were coloured with a brown eyeshadow using a dampened eyebrow brush.

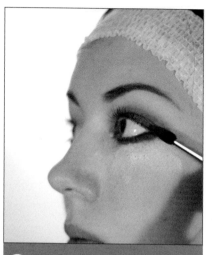

2 A base colour was applied from the lids to the brows. Then, using a dark black/brown to create a smoky eye a half-moon shape was applied to the eyelid. Some of the same colour was applied under the lower lashes. All the eyeshadow was blended using a cotton bud.

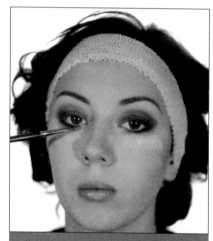

3 A silver shimmery eyeshadow was applied to the inside corner of the upper and lower lid avoiding the dark eyeshadow on the rest of the eyelid.

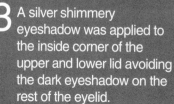

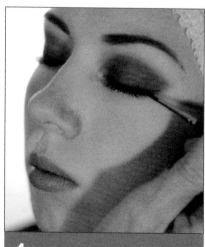

4 Using a thin pointed brush, eyeliner was applied close to the upper lashes. Mascara was then applied to the lashes.

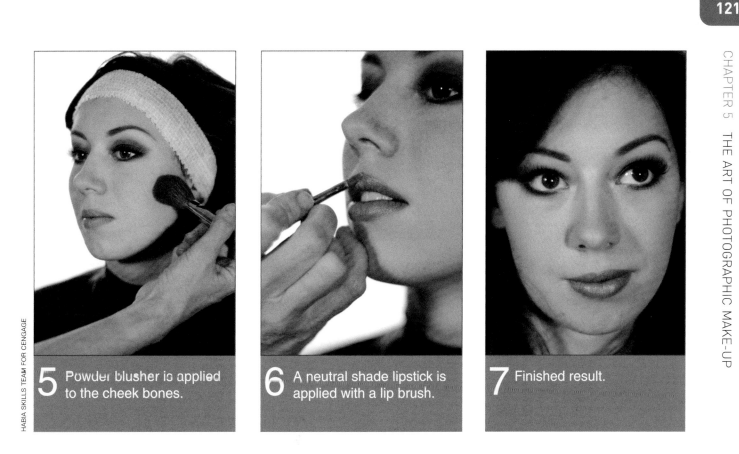

HABIA SKILLS TEAM FOR CENGAGE

5 Powder blusher is applied to the cheek bones.

6 A neutral shade lipstick is applied with a lip brush.

7 Finished result.

Photographic make-up (black and white)

The make-up for a black and white photograph requires strong colours. The make-up used for the previous step-by-step was enhanced. The eyelids were darkened using a black kohl pencil. A grey shader was applied under the cheekbones and a highlighter above the cheekbones. The lips were outlined using a dark plum lip pencil and coloured with the same colour lipstick.

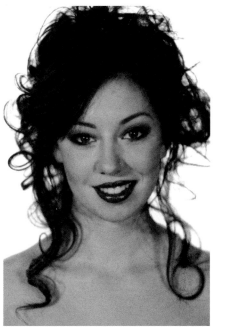

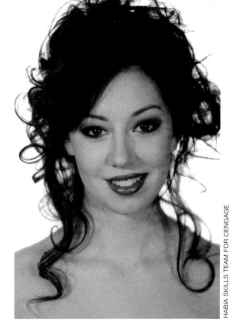

HABIA SKILLS TEAM FOR CENGAGE

Finished result in colour

Finished result in black and white

Providing aftercare advice

You may need to provide some advice to your model about how to look after their make-up. For example, if the make-up has been completed for a special occasion, such as a wedding, the make-up needs to last through the day and into the evening. Some brides engage a make-up artist who will return to freshen up the make-up for an evening reception. The bride should have a lipstick and gloss to match that applied by the make-up artist. Some make-up artists will provide the products to refresh the lips as part of their service.

If you are applying a make-up where you will remain with your model, you need to keep some make-up handy for touching up or refreshing the make-up. The lighting that the photographer will use is often very bright. Have some powder with you to prevent excessive light reflection from the skin. You may be asked to refresh the lip colour or tidy up the make-up several times, especially if your model is required to change their clothing for different pictures.

How to evaluate the effectiveness of the make-up application

It is important to reflect on the work you have completed. The skills you learn for the hair and beauty industries can never be perfected. You will always be improving.

When evaluating your work you could ask the following questions:

- Did the finished result meet the needs of my client?
- Did I work hygienically throughout the make-up application?
- Did I use the products correctly?
- What could I have done better?
- What did I do well?

You could ask these questions to yourself, or you could ask others who may have been working in your team. The client will also be able to provide feedback for you.

If you think there are areas you can improve on, make a plan for further training to improve your skills.

The work of a photographic make-up artist

Now that you have read this chapter, do you feel inspired? Would you like to be a photographic make-up artist?

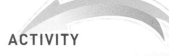

ACTIVITY

Research some photographic make-up artists – examine their portfolio of work. Many have their own websites to promote themselves and the work they have done. Have any of them completed any work that has really inspired you to study this subject further? Write a short report about your favourites and insert some images of their work into your report.

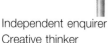

SIGNPOST PLTS

Independent enquirer
Creative thinker

TOP TIP

Put 'photographic make-up artist' into a search engine – you will find many examples.

SIGNPOST FUNCTIONAL SKILL

ICT

Use the internet to investigate some photographic make-up artists. When you do this, you will:

E3 use simple searches to find web-based sources of information

L1 use search techniques to locate and select relevant information.

English

Calculate the total costs to buy the tools, products and equipment for a self-employed photographic make-up artist. When you do this, you will:

E3   plan, draft and organize writing; sequence writing logically and clearly

L1   present information in a logical sequence. Write clearly and coherently, including an appropriate level of detail.

SIGNPOST FUNCTIONAL SKILL

What you have learnt

The importance of the preparation procedures for photographic make-up:

- The make-up application may not take place in the salon.
- You will have to be prepared to transport your kit.
- Your 'client' may not be the person you are working on.
- Carry out a consultation before you apply the make-up.
- Find out what the final result must look like.
- Ensure you have a good working space.
- Be prepared with a range of products for different looks.

The safe and hygienic procedures that must be followed:

- Ensure the area you are working in is safe and well lit.
- Work hygienically:
  - Do not 'double dip' your tools into make-up.
  - Prevent cross-infection.

How to select and use products, tools and equipment for photographic make-up application:

- Have a suitable range of make-up for different looks and racial skin tones.
- Use the correct brush to achieve a flawless finish for your photographic make-up.

The factors that affect photographic make-up application:

- Purpose:
  - Find out what the purpose of the make-up application is.
  - Have a consultation with your client, or attend a planning meeting.
  - Take notes and sketches to remind you about the meeting.
- Light:
  - Have sufficient light to apply the make-up in.
  - Check the finished result under the lights of the photographer.
  - Be prepared to adjust the make-up for different light conditions.

WHAT'S NEXT?

Technology for film and television is getting better all the time. **High definition** means that even the slightest flaw in a make-up application will be seen. Many make-up artists now do further training to specialize in **airbrushing** techniques for make-up application.

WHAT'S NEXT?

While photographic make-up is seen as very high fashion, some make-up artists like to improve the day-to-day lives of people affected with skin conditions they are born with or develop. For example, differences in skin tone, birth marks or scarring can be disguised with the clever use of make-up. With the application of **camouflage make-up**, such people can often feel more confident about their personal appearance.

- Colour:
  - ○ Find out which colours you will have to use.
  - ○ Prepare a mood board to show others how the end result will look.
- Time:
  - ○ Find out how much time you have to complete your make-up application.
  - ○ Find out how many models you will be working on.
  - ○ Plan your time carefully so that you don't get behind.
- Finished result:
  - ○ Find out if the finished result be in colour or black and white.
  - ○ Apply the make-up to ensure the finished result meets the requirements of your client.

The sequence in which make-up products should be applied:

- Have a look at the step-by-step images for a photographic make-up.

Providing aftercare advice:

- Be prepared to freshen up the make-up ready for the photographs to be taken.
- Provide clients with products in case they have to refresh their own make-up.
- Keep some face powder handy to prevent the skin reflecting too much light.

How to evaluate the effectiveness of the make-up application:

- Ask yourself:
  - ○ Did the finished result meet the needs of my client?
  - ○ Did I work hygienically throughout the make-up application?
  - ○ Did I use the products correctly?
  - ○ What could I have done better?
  - ○ What did I do well?

The work of a photographic make-up artist:

- Use the internet to investigate the work of photographic make-up artists.

ASSESSMENT ACTIVITIES

Activity 1 E3 – L1

These are short answer questions. Read the question carefully and then write down the answer.

1   You may have to transport your make-up kit to places outside the salon. How will you carry it?

2   Give **two** examples of the types of work you might do as a photographic make-up artist.

3   Describe what a brief is in relation to photographic make-up.

4   Give **three** examples for safe and hygienic working practices.

5   State why time is an important factor when applying photographic make-up.

Activity 2 E1 – L1

Place the sentences below into the correct order for applying photographic make-up on a bride.

Colour the eyebrows.

Apply eyeshadow.

Apply powder.

Cleanse, tone and moisturize.

Apply foundation.

Apply mascara.

Confirm the client is happy with the finished result.

Use concealer.

Apply lip colour.

Apply cream blusher.

1	
2	
3	
4	
5	
6	
7	
8	
9	
10	

Activity 3 E3–L1

Match the brush

Look at the images of the different types of make-up brush you can see in the first column of the table. In the second column read the list of why the brushes would be used. Draw an arrow from a purpose for use to the correct make-up brush.

Brush	Purpose for use
WWW.LOUISEYOUNGCOSMETICS.COM	To apply concealer to dark circles around the eye or to spots or blemishes.
WWW.LOUISEYOUNGCOSMETICS.COM	For the application of liquid and cream foundations.
WWW.LOUISEYOUNGCOSMETICS.COM	For applying and removing excess powder.
WWW.LOUISEYOUNGCOSMETICS.COM	For the application of blusher and for highlighting and contouring.

Brush	Purpose for use
WWW.LOUISEYOUNGCOSMETICS.COM	For applying and blending colours to the eyelids.
WWW.LOUISEYOUNGCOSMETICS.COM	For the precise application of eyeliner to the upper and lower lids.
WWW.LOUISEYOUNGCOSMETICS.COM	For the application of eyebrow products.
WWW.LOUISEYOUNGCOSMETICS.COM	For the application of lipstick and for blending lip liner.

6

Hand care and basic manicure nail art and pedicure

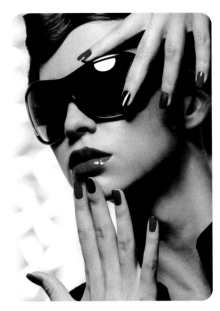

I am passionate about nails and know how vital it is they look groomed in today's society.

LEIGHTON DENNY, WINNER BRITISH NAIL TECHNICIAN OF THE YEAR 2001–04
AND VOTED INTO THE HALL OF FAME

In this chapter you are going to learn about:

- Importance of good hand and foot care.

- Nail structure and nail shapes.

- Selecting tools, products and equipment for manicure and pedicure treatments.

- Identifying the factors that affect hand and nail treatments and services.

- Preparing for and carrying out a hand treatment.

- Preparing for and carrying out a basic manicure.

- Preparing for and carrying out a basic pedicure.

- Preparing for and carrying out a nail art service.

- Designing a 2D image for nail art and adapting for a 3D surface.

Introduction

Looking after our hands and feet is very important; they work very hard for us all day. What would you do without them? **Manicures** and **pedicures** are very popular salon treatments because people like to have nice looking hands and feet. Not only do they like their hands and feet to look good but they also want the nails to be well presented. Fingernails and toenails can often be used to provide us with information of a person's individuality, especially through the use of nail art.

In this chapter you will learn how to help develop technical skills in carrying out basic manicure and pedicure treatments. You will also have the opportunity to use your artistic skills by designing a nail art image that you can then apply to a person's nail.

Importance of good hand and foot care

People say they can tell a lot about a person by their hands and feet. Some people's hands may look as though they do a lot of physical work, such as a builder or gardener, because their hands look dry, rough and uncared for. Other people may be nervous and take it out on their hands and feet by picking at them making them red and sore, or chewing their fingernails.

Looking at the condition of a person's hands and feet does not give you the full story of someone's life, but it's a start. You don't always need to have long painted fingernails to look good, but you do need to have nails that suit your lifestyle and provide a positive image about you.

IT'S A FACT!

A manicure involves the care of the hands and fingernails.

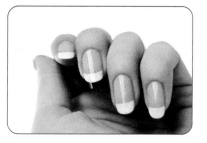

Having well-cared-for hands and nails gives a good first impression

ACTIVITY

This can be a group activity.

You can tell a lot about a person from their hands and nails. Discuss what you think about the appearance of the nails in photograph A and photograph B.

Photograph A

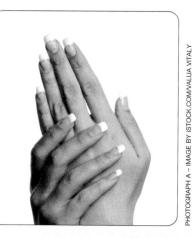

Photograph B

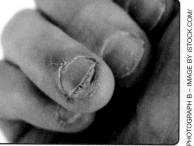

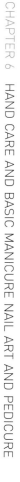

Discuss the following:

- What do you think the person would be like who has the nails in photograph A?

- What do you think the person would be like who has the nails in photograph B?

- Do you think that there would be situations when the person in photograph A would be limited in what they could do?

- Do you think that there would be situations when the person with the nails in photograph B may not want others to see them?

SIGNPOST PLTS

Teamwork
Creative thinker

SIGNPOST FUNCTIONAL SKILLS

English

When you discuss the differences in the two photographs, you will:

E3 respond appropriately to others and make some extended contributions in familiar formal or informal discussions and exchanges

L1 take full part in formal or informal discussions and exchanges that include unfamiliar subjects.

As well as a person's lifestyle, health can also be reflected in the condition of nails.

Nail structure

Nails are found at the end of your fingers and toes. They are there as a form of protection. You can also use your nails, particularly on your fingers, to pick up small, delicate objects.

The nail is made up of three main parts:

- Nail bed.
- Matrix.
- Nail plate.

Nail bed

- The nail bed is the living skin on which the nail plate sits.

- The nail bed is supplied with blood that gives the nail plate a pinkish appearance.

- The nail bed is supplied with **nerves**, so that you can feel pain.

- The nail bed is attached to a thin layer of tissue that acts as a seal against infection and also helps guide the nail along the nail bed as it grows.

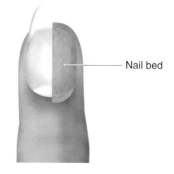

Nails can reflect your personality and lifestyle

IT'S A FACT!

Nails are made from **keratin**. This is the same protein that hair and skin is made from.

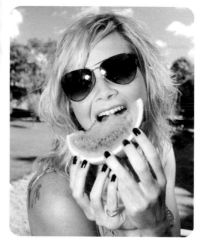

Nail bed

The nail bed

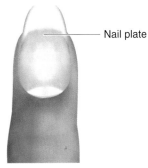

The matrix

The nail plate

Matrix

- The matrix is where the nail plate is formed.

- The part of the matrix you can see is called the **lunula.** This is the curve or half moon shape at the base of the nail that is a lighter colour than the rest of the nail plate.

Nail plate

- The nail plate is the visible and functional part of the nail.

- The nail plate is made from a hard keratin.

- The section of the nail plate that extends past the nail bed is called the **free edge**.

- Around the edge of the nail plate is a dead colourless tissue called the **cuticle**.

- The cuticle seals the space between the nail plate and living skin to prevent any infection or **micro-organisms** entering.

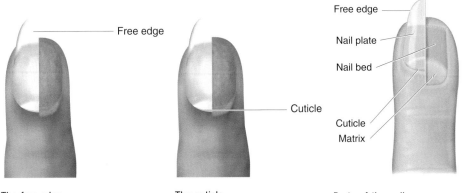

The free edge

The cuticle

Parts of the nail

WHAT'S NEXT?

When you study the nail structure as part of a Level 2 nail or beauty qualification, you will learn more about the structure of the hands, feet and nails. You will learn about the bone structure and the different muscles in the hands and feet that help support and enable them to move.

Nail shapes

When having a manicure or pedicure the nail can be shaped in different ways. As a professional beauty therapist or nail technician you will learn all about the different nail shapes and when to use them, to ensure that the finished nail will suit the shape and length of the client's hand or foot.

The advantages and disadvantages of different nail shapes:

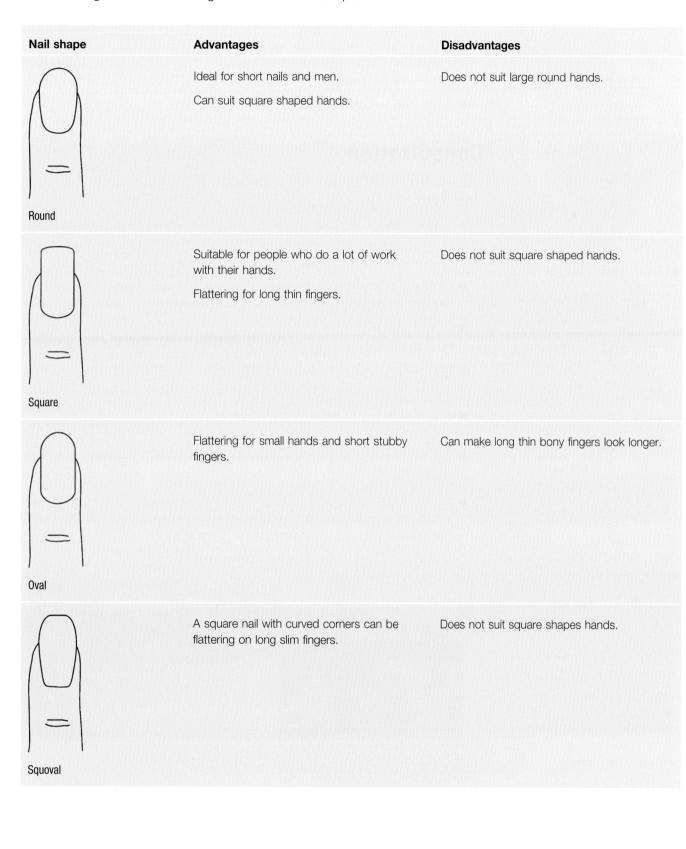

Nail shape	Advantages	Disadvantages
Round	Ideal for short nails and men. Can suit square shaped hands.	Does not suit large round hands.
Square	Suitable for people who do a lot of work with their hands. Flattering for long thin fingers.	Does not suit square shaped hands.
Oval	Flattering for small hands and short stubby fingers.	Can make long thin bony fingers look longer.
Squoval	A square nail with curved corners can be flattering on long slim fingers.	Does not suit square shapes hands.

IT'S A FACT!

Nails grow faster:

- On hands rather than feet.
- In children rather than older people.
- In summer rather than winter.

Nail growth

- Your nails grow on average 3.7 mm per month.
- Your nail growth can be affected by what you eat and your health.
- If you lose a fingernail it will take between 4 and 6 months to replace.
- If you lose a toenail it will take between 9 and 12 months to replace.

Consultation

You will always need to carry out a consultation prior to carrying out a manicure or pedicure.

There are certain factors that may affect your manicure or pedicure service and you will need to consider these before you carry out a service. As part of your consultation with the client you will need to discuss the following factors:

- Occasion: The look of the nails must be right for the occasion, for example the client may be going to a wedding or on holiday.
- Lifestyle: Work in certain professions will mean that fingernails will need to be short or they may not be able to wear nail enamel.
- Skin condition/type: If the skin is dry this will also affect the condition of the nail and cuticle. This could make the nail start to peel in layers.
- Allergies: Some clients may be allergic to ingredients that are in skin and nail products such as perfume in hand lotions.
- Nail shape: To ensure the finished nail will suit the shape and length of your client's hands.
- Skin and nail conditions that may affect the manicure or pedicure service: There are some diseases and disorders which mean that a service must not take place because the infection could be passed on to another person.

Hand, foot and nail diseases can include:

Viral condition

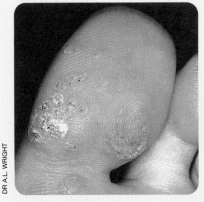

DR A.L. WRIGHT

Verruca

Verrucas grow into the skin and usually have black spots in the centre. They are found on the feet.

Bacterial condition

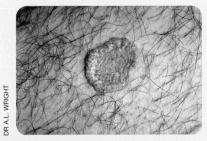

DR A.L. WRIGHT

Boils or furuncles

Furuncles are red painful swellings with a hard pus-filled core that goes down into the skin. Boils are formed around the hair follicles and can be found on the wrist.

Fungal conditions

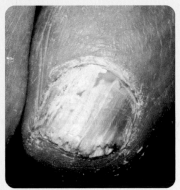

WELLCOME IMAGES

Ringworm of the nail plate

The nail plate will become yellowish-grey in colour, the nail plate will become dry and brittle and eventually separate from the nail bed.

Parasitic condition

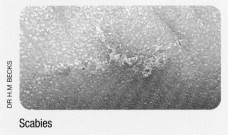

DR H.M BECKS

Scabies

A condition caused by an itchy mite which burrows through the skin, leaving greyish lines and reddish spots.

There are certain conditions that don't have to stop the total service but do restrict what you can do as part of the manicure or pedicure service. These include:

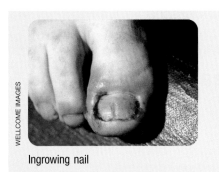

WELLCOME IMAGES

Ingrowing nail

This is a painful condition where the nail grows into the side of the nail bed creating pressure and swelling.

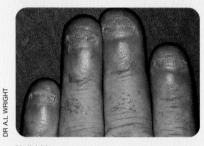

Areas of hard skin usually found on the top or sides of the toe. They are caused by pressure from ill-fitting shoes.

DR A.L WRIGHT

Corns

The free edge is often tender and the cuticles may be also bitten.

DR A.L WRIGHT

Nail biting

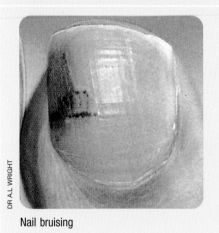

Damagie to the toenail by stubbing the toe or dropping something on it.

DR A.L WRIGHT

Nail bruising

WHAT'S NEXT?

When you study the nails as part of a Level 2 nail or beauty qualification, you will learn more about all the different types of skin and nail condition and disease that will affect a nail service.

As part of the consultation, after completing the analysis and recording the relevant information on a client record card, a professional will always complete a treatment plan.

Preparing the work area for a basic manicure or pedicure

When preparing your work area for a basic manicure for your client, you will need to make sure that the environment is comfortable and that the room area is ready with all the tools, materials, equipment and products you will be using. It is important to make sure that all the tools and equipment have been cleaned, disinfected or sterilized and that you always follow health and safety practices.

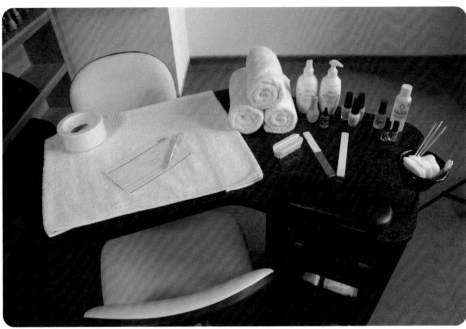

A prepared manicure table

A professional beauty therapist or nail technician will always make sure everything is ready for the client and the service.

Equipment, tools, products and materials checklist for a basic nail service

		Hand	Foot
Manicure table	Manicure/pedicure station or trolley on which to place everything	☐	☐
Towels	Medium sized towels: three for manicure, five for pedicure	☐	☐
	Small bowls lined with tissue (3) for clean cotton wool and putting products into	☐	☐

	Hand	Foot
Cotton wool — Dry cotton wool to apply and remove products from the skin and nails i.e. to apply nail polish remover to remove nail polish from the nails	☐	☐
Manicure bowl — Manicure bowl for the client's fingers – to cleanse the skin and nails and soften the skin in warm water	☐	
Pedicure spa — Pedicure bowl or spa for the client's feet – to cleanse the skin and nails and soften the skin in warm water		☐
Emery boards — Emery board to file the nail free edge to shape	☐	☐
Orange sticks — Orange sticks, tipped at either end with cotton wool, to apply products to the nails and to clean the nail on and around the nail plate. To gently loosen the cuticle. To remove products hygienically from their containers	☐	☐
Nail scissors — Nail scissors used to reduce the length of the nails before filing	☐	

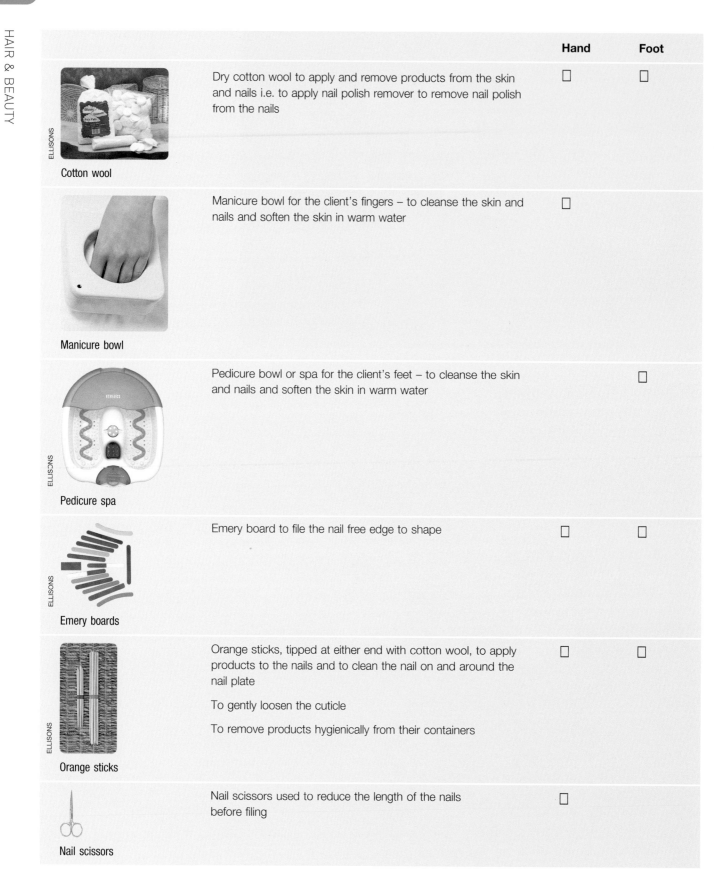

		Hand	Foot
Toenail clippers	Toenail clippers to shorten the length of the toenails		☐
Buffer	Buffers to give the nail a sheen improve the appearance of ridges when used with a buffing paste and to increase blood circulation to the nail	☐	☐
Buffing paste	Buffing paste, a course gritty nail product used to shine the nail plate when used with the buffer	☐	☐
ELLISONS
Detergent	Detergent, to add to the warm water in the manicure bowl or pedicure spa to cleanse and refresh the skin	☐	☐
SALON SYSTEMS
Hand cream	Hand cream, oil or lotion to soften and nourish the skin	☐	
SALON SYSTEMS
Foot cream | Foot cream, oil or lotion to soften and nourish the skin | | ☐ |

HAIR & BEAUTY

		Hand	Foot

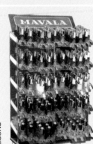
Skin sanitizer

Skin sanitizer to cleanse the skin before the service

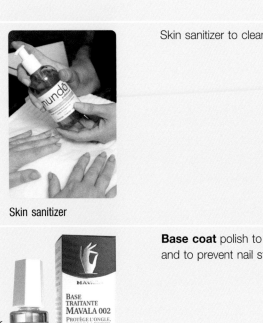
Base coat

Base coat polish to provide a base to apply coloured polish and to prevent nail staining

Light coloured polishes

Light coloured polishes, a selection

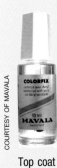
Top coat

Top coat to seal and protect nail polish colour providing durability

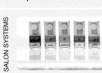
Nail strengthener

Specialist nail products such a nail strengthener

COURTESY OF MAVALA

ELLISONS

COURTESY OF MAVALA

SALON SYSTEMS

			Hand	Foot
Nail polish remover		Nail polish remover, to remove nail polish from the nail	☐	☐
Cuticle oil		Cuticle oil to soften and nourish the skin of the cuticle	☐	☐
Cuticle massage cream		Cuticle massage cream to soften and nourish the skin of the cuticle	☐	☐
Disinfectant solution		Small jar of disinfecting solution to hold small metal and plastic nail service tools	☐	☐
Metal bin		Metal bin – lined with a disposable bin liner	☐	☐

CREATIVE NAILS

IT'S A FACT!

A pedicure involves the care of the feet and toenails.

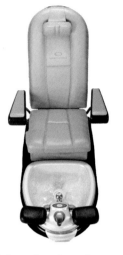

Work station set-up for pedicure.

	Hand	Foot
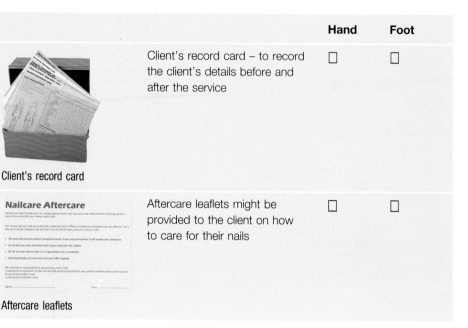 Client's record card	Client's record card – to record the client's details before and after the service	☐	☐
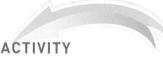 Aftercare leaflets	Aftercare leaflets might be provided to the client on how to care for their nails	☐	☐

TOP TIP

Nail enamel peels if:

- It is applied too quickly.
- Poor quality or thickened nail enamel is used.
- Oil or grease is left on the nail plate.

ACTIVITY

Why not find out a bit more about nail products and manicure procedures. Use the internet to look for more information. You can try the websites listed below:

http://www.millenniumnailsonline.com
http://www.opi.com
http://www.mavala.com

Identify the different types of product and what they are used for. Make an information leaflet that you can give to clients to tell them about the products.

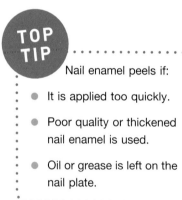

SIGNPOST FUNCTIONAL SKILLS

SIGNPOST PLTS

Independent enquirer
Creative thinker

ICT

When you are looking at websites for information on nail products and manicure procedures you will interact with ICT for a given purpose and you will be able to recognize and use interface features. **E3** and **L1**

When you read the information on the website about the styling and finishing products, you will:

E3 and **L1** read and understand the purpose and context of straightforward texts.

When you write about the styling and finishing products, you will:

E3 plan, draft and organize your writing and write logically and clearly checking your grammar, punctuation and spelling

L1 write logically and clearly including an appropriate level of details. You will use the correct grammar ensuring the accurate punctuation and spelling.

Massage techniques used in a basic manicure and pedicure

As part of any service you will need to carry out basic massage strokes. There are three main groups of massage movement. The table below lists the main movements in each of the three groups:

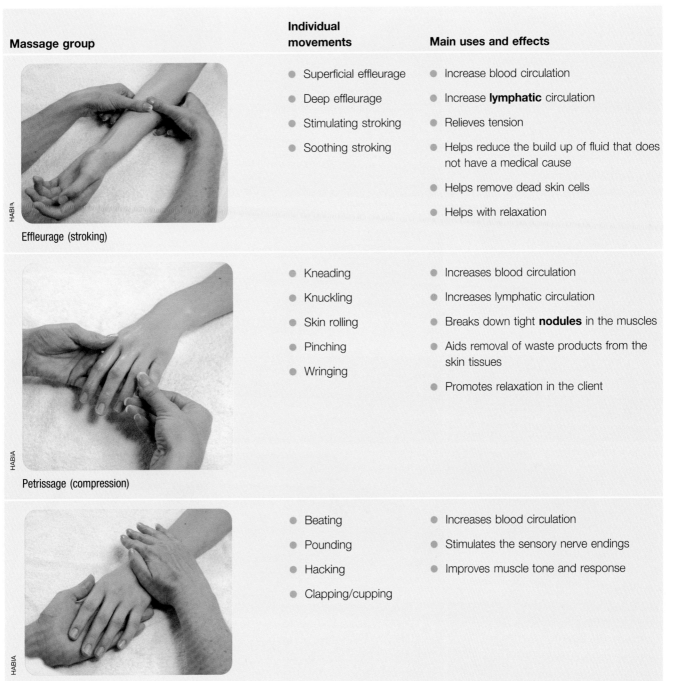

Massage group	Individual movements	Main uses and effects
Effleurage (stroking)	• Superficial effleurage • Deep effleurage • Stimulating stroking • Soothing stroking	• Increase blood circulation • Increase **lymphatic** circulation • Relieves tension • Helps reduce the build up of fluid that does not have a medical cause • Helps remove dead skin cells • Helps with relaxation
Petrissage (compression)	• Kneading • Knuckling • Skin rolling • Pinching • Wringing	• Increases blood circulation • Increases lymphatic circulation • Breaks down tight **nodules** in the muscles • Aids removal of waste products from the skin tissues • Promotes relaxation in the client
Tapotement (percussion)	• Beating • Pounding • Hacking • Clapping/cupping	• Increases blood circulation • Stimulates the sensory nerve endings • Improves muscle tone and response

Carrying out a basic manicure

Step-by-step method for a basic manicure procedure

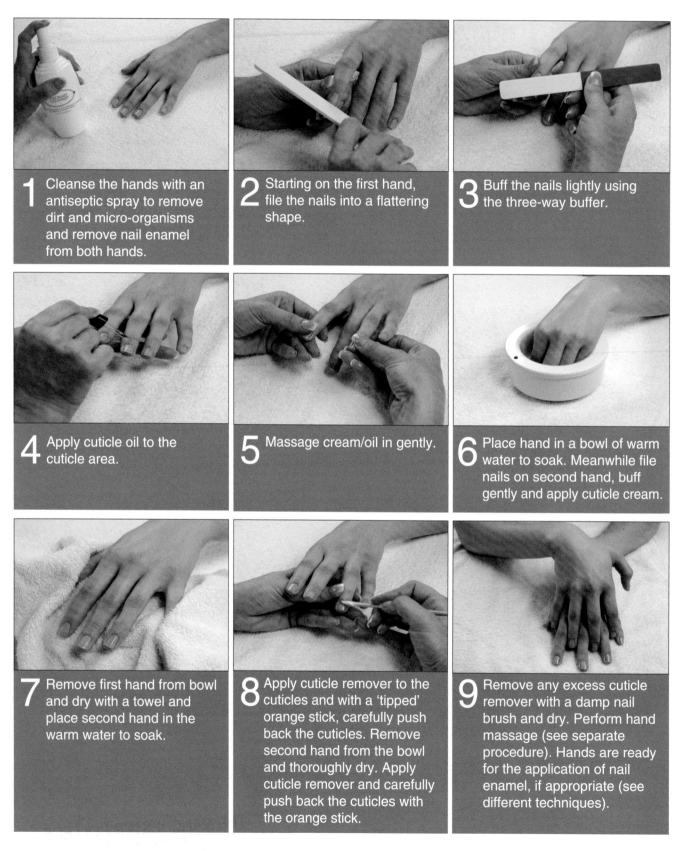

1 Cleanse the hands with an antiseptic spray to remove dirt and micro-organisms and remove nail enamel from both hands.

2 Starting on the first hand, file the nails into a flattering shape.

3 Buff the nails lightly using the three-way buffer.

4 Apply cuticle oil to the cuticle area.

5 Massage cream/oil in gently.

6 Place hand in a bowl of warm water to soak. Meanwhile file nails on second hand, buff gently and apply cuticle cream.

7 Remove first hand from bowl and dry with a towel and place second hand in the warm water to soak.

8 Apply cuticle remover to the cuticles and with a 'tipped' orange stick, carefully push back the cuticles. Remove second hand from the bowl and thoroughly dry. Apply cuticle remover and carefully push back the cuticles with the orange stick.

9 Remove any excess cuticle remover with a damp nail brush and dry. Perform hand massage (see separate procedure). Hands are ready for the application of nail enamel, if appropriate (see different techniques).

Carrying out a hand massage

Step-by-step method for a hand massage procedure

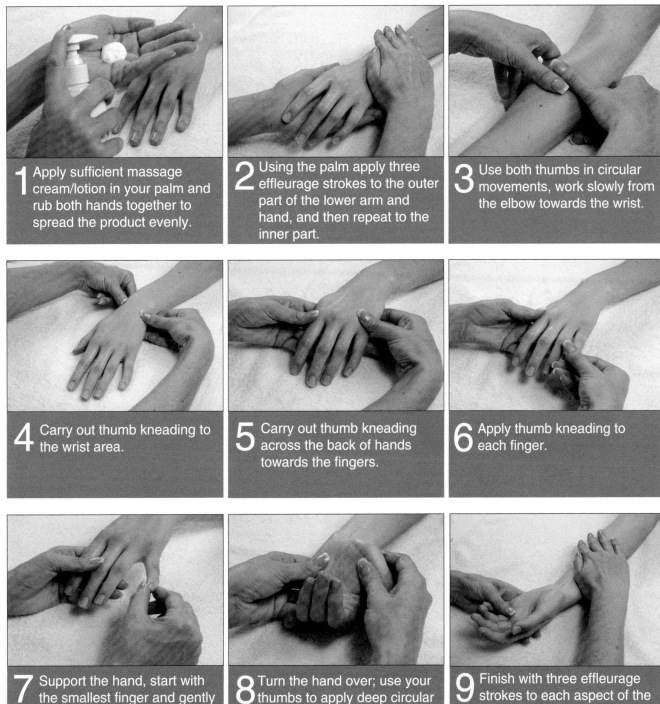

1 Apply sufficient massage cream/lotion in your palm and rub both hands together to spread the product evenly.

2 Using the palm apply three effleurage strokes to the outer part of the lower arm and hand, and then repeat to the inner part.

3 Use both thumbs in circular movements, work slowly from the elbow towards the wrist.

4 Carry out thumb kneading to the wrist area.

5 Carry out thumb kneading across the back of hands towards the fingers.

6 Apply thumb kneading to each finger.

7 Support the hand, start with the smallest finger and gently rotate each finger twice in each direction. Finish with a slight pull, and a sliding motion off the end of the finger.

8 Turn the hand over; use your thumbs to apply deep circular kneading movements across the whole palm area, paying particular attention to the base of the thumb.

9 Finish with three effleurage strokes to each aspect of the lower arm and hand.

TOP TIP

Advise your clients to wear open-toed sandals when coming for a pedicure to allow time for the nail enamel to dry completely and avoid smudging.

IT'S A FACT!

The word pedicure comes from the Latin words *pedis*, meaning foot, and *cura*, meaning care.

Correct nail enamel application

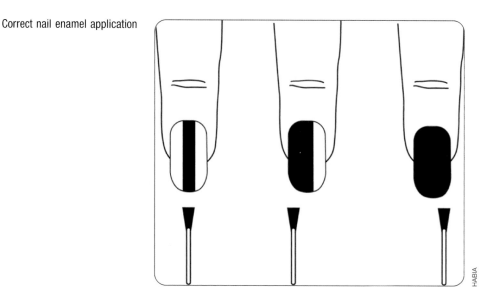

Carrying out a basic pedicure

Step-by-step method for a pedicure procedure

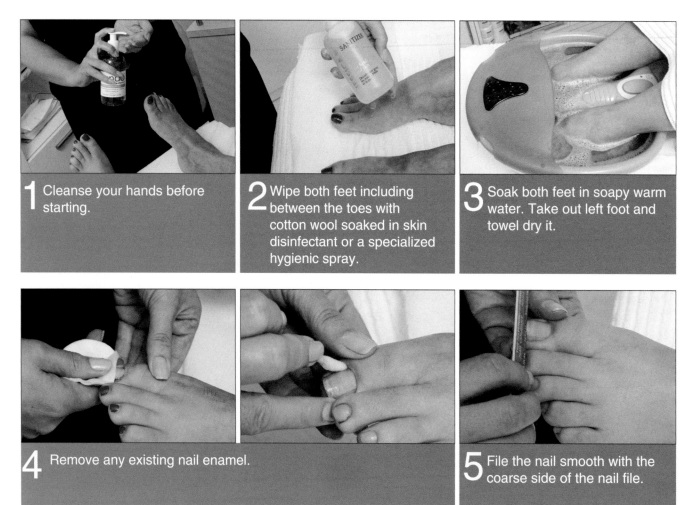

1 Cleanse your hands before starting.

2 Wipe both feet including between the toes with cotton wool soaked in skin disinfectant or a specialized hygienic spray.

3 Soak both feet in soapy warm water. Take out left foot and towel dry it.

4 Remove any existing nail enamel.

5 File the nail smooth with the coarse side of the nail file.

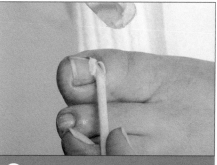

6 Apply cuticle cream or oil. Place the foot back in the water to soften the cuticle. Remove the right foot from the water and repeat steps 3 to 6.

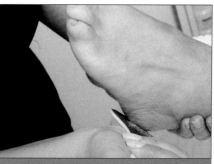

7 Take out the left foot and towel dry it. Remove any hard skin by using either a file /rasp or exfoliating cream. Put the left foot back into the water to remove exfoliating cream if used, and repeat on the right foot.

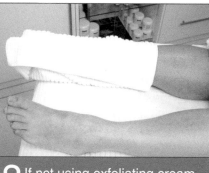

8 If not using exfoliating cream wrap the foot in a dry towel to keep it warm while working on the other foot. Remove the foot bowl from the work area after use.

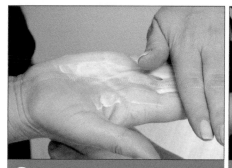

9 You can now carry out a simple foot and lower leg massage. Apply massage cream/oil into the hands and apply to your client's skin using effleurage movements.

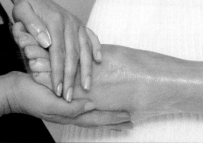
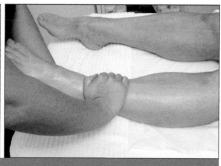

10 Effleurage from the foot to the knee. Use long sweeping strokes from the toes to the knee, moving on both the back and the front of the leg. Repeat on the other leg.

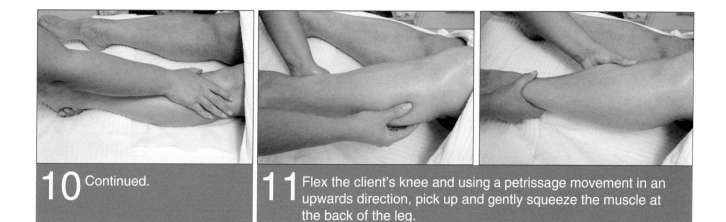

10 Continued.

11 Flex the client's knee and using a petrissage movement in an upwards direction, pick up and gently squeeze the muscle at the back of the leg.

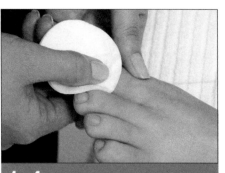

12 Using the pads of the fingers use small circular kneading movements around the ankle bone.

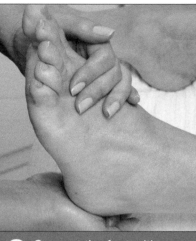

13 Support the foot with one hand and using the palm cup the heel and perform a circular kneading movement. Repeat on the other foot.

14 Remove any grease from the nail plates with a cotton wool pad soaked in nail polish remover. Refile the nails as necessary to ensure they are smooth and even.

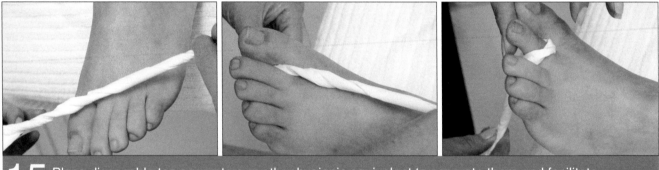

15 Place disposable toe separators or other hygienic equivalent to separate them and facilitate polish application.

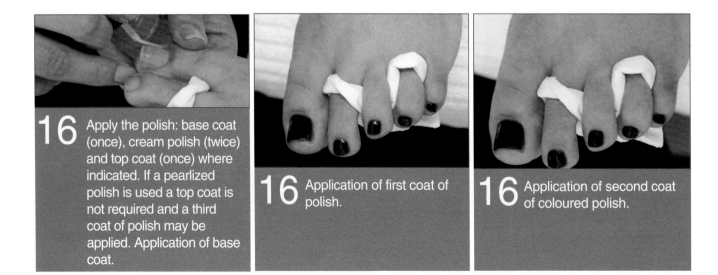

16 Apply the polish: base coat (once), cream polish (twice) and top coat (once) where indicated. If a pearlized polish is used a top coat is not required and a third coat of polish may be applied. Application of base coat.

16 Application of first coat of polish.

16 Application of second coat of coloured polish.

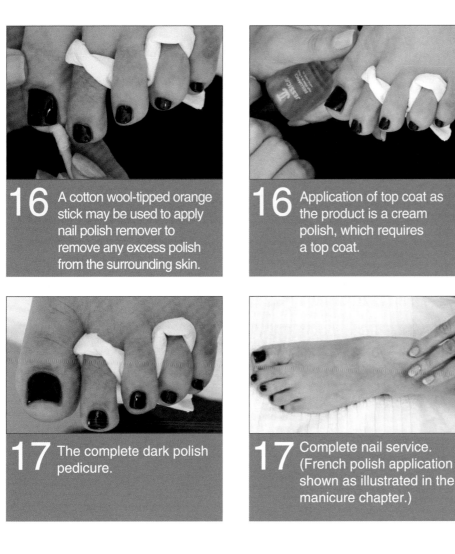

16 A cotton wool-tipped orange stick may be used to apply nail polish remover to remove any excess polish from the surrounding skin.

16 Application of top coat as the product is a cream polish, which requires a top coat.

17 The complete dark polish pedicure.

17 Complete nail service. (French polish application shown as illustrated in the manicure chapter.)

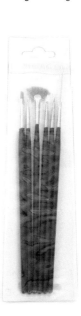

STAR NAILS

Dotting/marbling tool

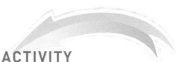

Nail art brushes

Nail art

To be good at nail art you need to be skilled at painting nails. You will need to practise a great deal and you will also need a steady hand, patience and skill.

Nail art has become very popular and you can see lots of people wearing nail art, including high profile celebrities.

To carry out nail art successfully you will need to use a set of nail art brushes. These will include:

- Flat brush: Small flat brush to create shading, smudging and swirls.
- Striping brush: Of different lengths and thicknesses so that you can produce stripes, lines and flicks.
- Detail brush: Small brush used for detail work such as small dots.

Specialist water-based acrylic paints are used. A base coat is applied to the nail then you can use a variety of nail art brushes and a marbling tool to create lots of different effects:

- Dots of colour.
- Marbling where you blend two or three colours.

ACTIVITY

Why not find out a bit more about nail art and the different designs that can be produced. Use the internet to look for more information. You can try the websites listed below to find different nail art images and video clips:

http://www.nailartgallery.com
http://www.thenaildirectory.com
http://www.creativeten.co.uk

SIGNPOST
PLTS

Independent enquirer

- Stripes across the corners of the nail or fanning out from one side.
- Stencils can be applied to the nail and then painted over.
- Pictures can be created or copied from a design.

You can get ideas for nail art designs from all sorts of things. Before you carry out any nail art it is best to draw the design on paper or follow a design that has already been produced. When you have a flat image of a design it is called a 2D image. When you transfer that design onto a nail it will become a 3D image.

SIGNPOST
FUNCTIONAL
SKILLS

ICT

When you are looking at websites for information on nail art you will interact with ICT for a given purpose and you will be able to recognize and use interface features. **E3** and **L1**

SIGNPOST
FUNCTIONAL
SKILLS

English

When you read the information on the website about nail art, you will:

E3 and **L1**   read and understand the purpose and context of straightforward texts.

SIGNPOST
PLTS

Creative thinker
Self-manager
Independent enquirer
Reflective learner

ACTIVITY

Produce a number of nail art designs that you could use to show your clients during the consultation process. The designs need to be carefully drawn and coloured so that the client can clearly see the detail of the design and they should look professional. Your designs could then be transferred onto an artificial nail to show them in 3D.

TOP TIP

Make sure the coats of nail enamel are touch dry before you start the nail art.

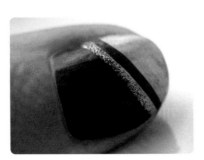

A simple stripe design can be achieved using tape or painted on

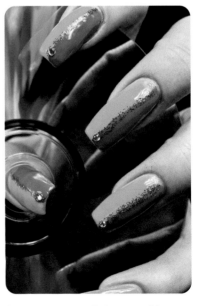

Simple nail art can look very striking

Nail art products and materials:

Products and materials	How to use them
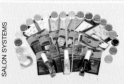 SALON SYSTEMS **Glitter enamels and dust**	Can be used in a variety of ways. Over the whole nail, on the free edge or on a specific part of the nail to highlight a design: ● Dip brush in sealer. ● Pick up the glitter on the end of the brush. ● Apply to nail. ● Secure the design with sealer, by carefully applying a thick coat to protect the glitter.
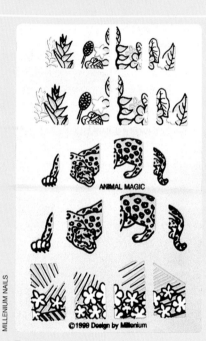 MILLENIUM NAILS **Transfers and tapes**	These are ready made for nail art: ● Some transfers peel off a backing and can be stuck straight onto the nail. ● Some transfers need soaking first, before sliding onto the nail. ● Tapes come in a variety of widths, colours and patterns. ● Tapes are sticky backed and can be trimmed once they are in place on the nail. ● A thick coat of sealer is applied to protect the design.
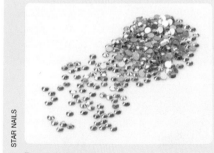 STAR NAILS **Enamel/polish secures**	Secures is the generic name given to a range of items that have a flat back and are used in nail art: ● Apply the nail enamel and top coat. ● Use an orange stick to pick up the secure and place them. ● Carefully place them on to wet nail enamel. ● They are then sealed to protect the design. Secures can include: ● Pearls. ● Beads. ● Stone shapes or flower shapes. ● Diamanté. ● Foils shapes such as stars, palm trees. ● Metal studs.

Applying a nail enamel with a transfer

Step-by-step method for applying a nail enamel with a transfer

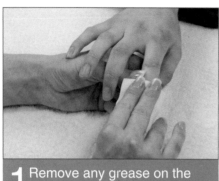

1 Remove any grease on the nail plate with the nail enamel remover.

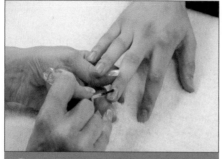

2 Select and apply the base coat.

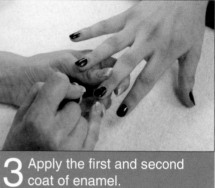

3 Apply the first and second coat of enamel.

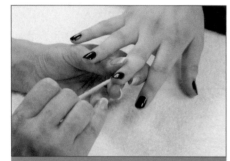

4 Tip an orange stick with cotton wool, wrap the cotton wool tightly around the orange stick, dip the tipped orange stick in enamel remover and remove any smudges of enamel, to ensure a perfect finish.

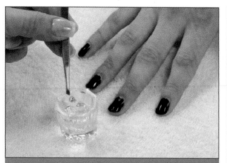

5 Select a nail transfer and soak it in water.

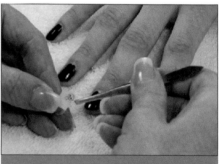

6 Use tweezers to slide the transfer from the backing paper.

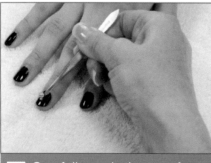

7 Carefully apply the transfer to the nail, and ensure the transfer is positioned carefully on the nail.

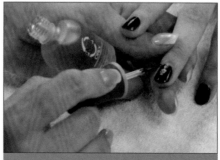

8 Apply a coat of top coat/sealer to protect the enamel, transfer and prolong the life of the manicure.

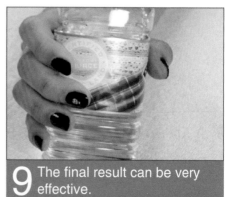

9 The final result can be very effective.

Blending technique

Step-by-step method for blending

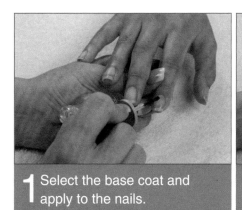

1 Select the base coat and apply to the nails.

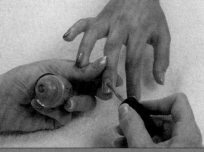

2 First apply the lightest colour all over the nail, making sure the colour is applied evenly.

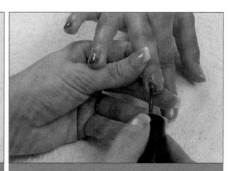

3 Apply the darker colour to the tip of the nail, creating a diagonal line. Ensure the dark colour is applied evenly.

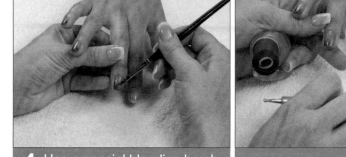

4 Use a special blending brush to blend the line between the two colours. Work quickly to ensure the colours blend easily.

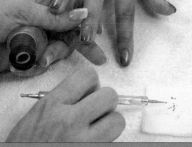

5 Prepare small glitter dots, place some on a tissue. Ensure you have the correct tool ready.

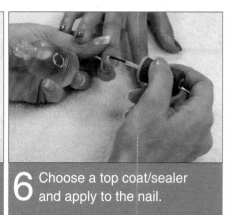

6 Choose a top coat/sealer and apply to the nail.

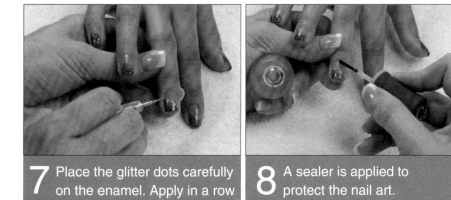

7 Place the glitter dots carefully on the enamel. Apply in a row along the blended line.

8 A sealer is applied to protect the nail art.

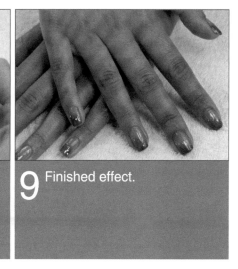

9 Finished effect.

Sterilizing tools and equipment

After you have completed a manicure or pedicure you need to make sure that you clean, disinfect or sterilize tools and equipment straight away, so that they are ready for use on the next client. Chapter 9, 'Safe and hygienic working practices' will give you guidance on sterilizing tools and equipment.

Remember a professional would never use dirty tools and equipment.

Aftercare

You will need to give aftercare advice to your client about how to look after their manicure or pedicure at home so that it lasts longer and the skin and nails stay in good condition. You can recommend products for them to use at home, to help continue the effects you have achieved.

What you have learnt

The importance of good hand and foot care:

- Hands, feet and nails can tell you a lot about a person.

The basic nail structure and nail shapes:

- Understanding the different parts of the nail.

That the nails are made up of a protein called keratin, which is also found in your hair and skin:

- The advantages and disadvantages of different nail shapes.

Selecting tools, products and equipment for manicure and pedicure treatments.

Identifying the factors that affect nail treatments and services:

- The different types of hand, foot and nail disorder and condition that can affect or restrict a service.

How to prepare for and carry out a hand or foot treatment.

The basic techniques for carrying out a basic manicure or pedicure.

The basic techniques for carrying out a nail art service.

ASSESSMENT ACTIVITIES

Activity 1 E3 and L1

Label the diagram

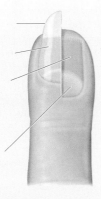

Activity 2 E3 and L1

Complete the following text by adding the correct word/s from the table into the missing spaces:

chewing	feet	hands	painted	red
condition	gardener	nails	physical	uncared

People say they can tell a lot about a person by their _____ and feet. Some people's hands may look like they do a lot of _____ work such as a builder or _____ because their hands look dry, rough and _____ for. Other people may be nervous and take it out on their hands and _____ by picking at them making them _____ and sore, or _____ their fingernails.

Looking at the _____ of a person's hands and feet does not give you the full story of someone's life, but it's a start. You don't always need to have long _____ fingernails to look good, but you do need to have _____ that suit your lifestyle and provide a positive image about you.

Activity 3 E3 and L1

Blockbuster

Work with a partner or split into two teams. Choose a letter and answer the question. When you have answered the question correctly, mark off the square. See who can correctly answer the questions to complete a straight or diagonal line across the grid. You can block the way of your partner or other team to stop them winning!

M	N	T	H	S
P	B	R	C	B
K	L	S	I	E
B	F	O	V	P
P	C	S	R	T

M	Which M is a service carried out on the hands? ____
P	Which P is a service carried out on the feet? _____
K	Which K is a protein that nails are made from? _____
B	Which B is one of the three main parts that make up the nail? _____
M	Which M is one of the three main parts that make up the nail? _____
P	Which P is one of the main three parts that make up the nail? _____
N	Which N enables use to feel pain? _____
B	Which B gives the nail plate a pinkish appearance? _____
L	Which L is part of the matrix that we can see? _____
F	Which F extends past the nail bed? _____
C	Which C seals the space between the nail plate and living skin? _____
T	Which T is used to describe a person that works with nails? _____
R	Which R is used to describe a nail shape? _____
S	Which S is a nail shape best suited for people that do a lot of work with their hands? _____
O	Which O is used to describe a nail shape? _____
S	Which S is a nail shape that is a mixture of square and oval? _____

H	Which H do nails grow faster on? _____
C	Which C is the name of the process you carry out before a service? _____
I	Which I do you find out as part of a consultation? _____
V	Which V is a viral condition found on the foot? _____
R	Which R is a fungal condition found on the nail plate? _____

S	Which S is a parasitic condition that leaves greyish lines and reddish spots on the skin? _____
B	Which B is a type of skin condition? _____
E	Which E is a type of massage movement? _____
P	Which P is a type of massage movement? _____
T	Which T is a type of massage movement? _____

Activity 4 E3 and L1

Link the boxes on the left with the appropriate boxes on the right. You may use different coloured markers to show your connections.

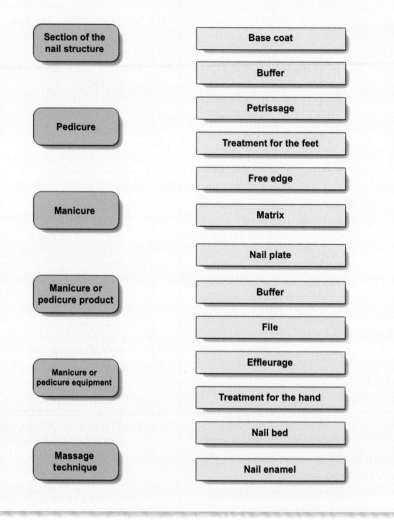

7
Introduction to hair care

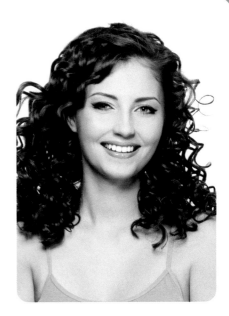

I'm undaunted in my quest to amuse myself by constantly changing my hair.

HILLARY CLINTON, AMERICAN POLITICIAN

In this chapter you are going to learn about:

- The basic structure of the hair.
- How to analyze your hair.
- How hair grows.
- Head and face shapes.
- How to prepare for hair care services.
- Shampooing and conditioning the hair.

Introduction

If you want to work in the hairdressing or barbering industry you have to know all about hair. You need to understand all about the hair structure and how to look after the hair of your clients. Your hair is a very important feature of your whole appearance. It is one of the first things that people will notice about you. The condition of your hair is also very important. You need to care for it if you want it to look nice. When you read this chapter you will learn all about how to care for your own hair and learn how to look after the hair of clients.

The basic structure of hair

Hair covers the whole of your body except the lips, palms of the hands and the soles of the feet. Hair is made of a protein called keratin. Your skin and nails are also made of keratin. You have different types of hair on different parts of your

IT'S A FACT!

Feathers and fur are also made from keratin.

IT'S A FACT!

Animals use their hair as a warning system. Have you noticed that if dogs or cats are frightened, their hair will stand out? And, sometimes, if you are alarmed you can feel your hairs on your neck stand on end.

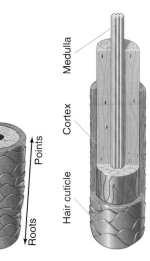

Hair structure showing three layers

IT'S A FACT!

The medulla is not always present in hair. Sometimes its place is taken by the cortex. You are less likely to have a medulla if your hair is fine.

ACTIVITY

You can tell the condition of your hair by feeling the cuticle. Work with a partner and hold a few strands of hair. Slide your thumb and first finger from the ends of the hair towards the roots. What do you feel? Does the hair feel rough or smooth? If it feels smooth it means that the cuticle is lying flat and the hair is in good condition. If it feels rough, the cuticle may be open. It may mean that the hair is not in good condition.

SIGNPOST PLTS

Teamworker
Creative thinker
Reflective learner

body. Some hair is soft and fine and known as **vellus hair**, other hair, such as the hair on your head or that on the beard of a man, is called **terminal hair**.

The function of hair is to protect your head and keep you warm. The hair on the body can also help to keep you warm. Have you noticed what happens when you are cold? The hairs stand up, trapping a layer of warm air. Other hair, such as your eyelashes, are used as a warning system. The fine hair will detect something that might otherwise go into your eye.

The sections of the hair

Each hair strand is made of up to three sections. The three sections of hair are called:

- Cuticle.
- Cortex.
- Medulla.

The cuticle

The cuticle is the outside layer of your hair. It is made up of overlapping scales rather like tiles on the roof of a house or like the bark of a tree. The number of layers of cuticle varies from one person to another. For example, if you have fine hair, you may only have three cuticle layers. But coarser hair can have up to 11 layers. The cuticle is translucent. This means that you can almost see through it into the next layer of hair, the cortex.

When hair is in good condition all the scales of the cuticle will lie flat with the free edge pointing towards the ends of the hair. If you have a flat surface, light is

ACTIVITY

Which of the cuticles are in good and poor condition?

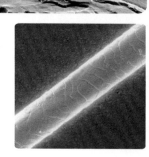

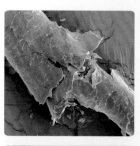

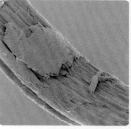

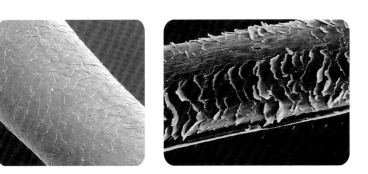

Close-up image of cuticle scales showing hair in good and poor condition

IT'S A FACT!

Hair is more likely to look shiny when it is straight. Light does not reflect so well from curly hair. However, this does not mean that the hair is not in good condition.

reflected from it. So when light is reflected from the surface of the hair, it looks shiny and healthy.

The function of the cuticle is to protect the inner layer of the hair called the cortex.

English

Do the porosity test activity on a number of different people and write down the results. When you do this, you will:

E3 plan, draft and organize writing; sequence writing logically and clearly

L1 present information in a logical sequence; write clearly and coherently, including an appropriate level of detail.

SIGNPOST FUNCTIONAL SKILL

The cortex

This layer makes up more than 90 per cent of the hair structure. Inside this layer are special bonds that give the hair its strength. The bonds form together to make coiled, ladder-like links that give hair its strength and elasticity. When hair is in good condition, it will stretch and then return to its normal length.

WHAT'S NEXT?

When you progress to Level 2 hair structure you will learn about how the condition of the cuticle will affect the way the hair is coloured. You will also learn that the test you have just completed for the activity is called a **porosity test**.

ACTIVITY

You can check the condition of your cortex by carrying out a test. Work with a partner and hold a single strand of their hair, supporting it at the roots to ensure you do not hurt them. Gently stretch the hair, and then release it. Look to see how soon it returns to its normal position. If the cortex is in good condition it will stretch and then go back to its normal position very quickly. If the cortex is not in very good condition, the hair may return to its normal position much more slowly. However, hair with a cortex that is in very poor condition may stretch and keep stretching. It may not return to its normal position. It may even break under the slightest pressure.

SIGNPOST PLTS

Independent enquirer

WHAT'S NEXT?

When you progress to Level 2 hairdressing or barbering you will learn about the names of the bonds in the hair, and how the condition of the cortex will affect the way the hair is straightened or permed. You will also learn that the test you have just completed for the activity is called an **elasticity test**.

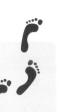

SIGNPOST PLTS

Teamworker
Creative thinker
Reflective learner

**SIGNPOST
FUNCTIONAL
SKILL**

SIGNPOST
PLTS

Independent enquirer

WHAT'S NEXT?

When you progress to Level 2 hair structure you will find out the names of all the special bonds that allow hair to stretch and return to its normal length. You will also learn about how the bonds are broken and join together again during styling, perming and straightening.

WEB LINK

You can download a pdf file from the Wella Professionals site called 'Interesting facts about the topic of hair'. In this document you will find images of hair that have been magnified. You will also find, on page 7, an image of the medulla. **http://www .wellaprofessionals.co.uk/ reference/to_download_ 5010_0_sl.pdf**

**SIGNPOST
FUNCTIONAL
SKILL**

SIGNPOST
PLTS

Independent enquirer

English
Do the elasticity test activity on a number of different people and write down the results. When you do this, you will: E3   plan, draft and organize writing; sequence writing logically and clearly L1   present information in a logical sequence; write clearly and coherently, including an appropriate level of detail.

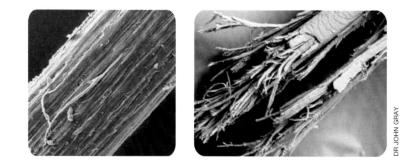

DR JOHN GRAY

Close up image of the cortex in good and poor condition

The cortex is a very important layer of hair. Within this layer you will find the cells that contain melanin. Melanin is the natural colour pigment of hair. You can see the natural colour of hair through the translucent layer of the cuticle. When hair is coloured some types of artificial colour will enter the cortex, which you can also see through the cuticle layer.

The medulla

The medulla is found in the centre of the hair. It is just an air space, sometimes filled with soft, spongy cells. Not all hair has a medulla. However, this does not matter as the medulla does not have a function and if missing its place is taken by the cortex.

ICT
When you look at the web link for the hair structure you will interact with ICT for a given purpose and you will be able to recognize and use interface features. **E1 – E3**

The appendages of hair

The appendages of the hair are found in the dermis of the skin. You will learn more about the dermis of the skin in Chapter 4, 'Skincare make-up and face painting'.

In the dermis of the skin you find the following appendages which are attached to or belong to the hair:

- Hair follicle.
- Arrector pili muscle.

- Sebaceous gland.
- Papilla.
- Blood supply.
- Nerves.

Hair follicle

The hair follicle is a thin tube in the skin. The hair grows inside the hair follicle and it holds the hair in place.

Arrector pili muscle

This is a muscle that is attached to the base of the hair follicle and the underside of the epidermis (which is the very top layer of the skin). When you are cold or frightened, the **arrector pili** muscle tightens, becoming shorter. This makes the hair stand up and causes goose bumps.

Sebaceous gland

This gland is attached to the hair follicle and produces the natural oil of the hair and skin. The oil is called sebum. The sebum passes onto the skin surface from the hair follicle.

Papilla

The papilla is found at the base of the hair follicle and is the place where all new hair cells are formed.

Blood supply

Blood enters the base of the follicle at the papilla to provide nutrients for the development of healthy hair cells.

Nerves

The hair itself does not have any nerves. That is why you cannot feel anything when the hair is cut. But there are nerves that surround the outside of the hair follicle. This is why you can feel your hair when it is moved.

Finding out about your hair

We all have different hair. It is different in the way that it looks, the way that it grows and even the way it feels.

To know all about your hair or that of clients, you have to analyze it. You need to analyze hair before you can carry out any hairdressing treatments and services. You need to consider the following:

- Hair type.
- Hair texture.
- Hair condition.

WEB LINK

Look at this web link from L'Oréal Science http://www.hair-science.com/_int/_en/topic/topic_sousrub.aspx?tc=ROOT-HAIR-SCIENCE^PORTRAIT-OF-AN-UNKNOWN-ELEMENT^WHAT-WE-DO-SEE&cur=WHAT-WE-DO-SEE. You can click into the image of the hair and see all the sections close up.

IT'S A FACT!

An appendage is something that is added onto, attached to or belongs to something else.

IT'S A FACT!
An image
The size of the follicle varies depending on the type of hair in it. The follicles on your arm will be shorter and thinner than those you have on your head.

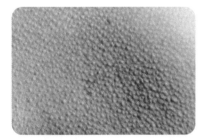

You get goose bumps when you are cold

IT'S A FACT!

An *overactive* sebaceous gland will make the skin and hair too oily. If you have an *underactive* sebaceous gland your hair and skin will be too dry.

- Hair density.
- Hair length.
- Hair growth patterns.

Hair type

Hair type is how curly or straight your hair is. There are three main hair types. They are:

- African.
- Asian.
- Caucasian.

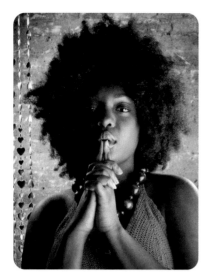

African type hair

African type hair This hair type is very curly, frizzy and woolly. The curls can also vary from very soft open curls to tightly closed curls. It is usually dark in colour, but can be anything from blonde to red.

Asian type hair Asian hair is usually very dark in colour. Oriental hair such as you can see in Japan is often very straight, whereas hair found in India and Pakistan can be wavier.

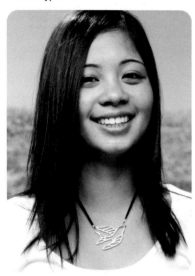

Asian type hair

Caucasian type hair This hair type, sometimes called European hair, can vary from very curly to very straight. It can be very dark or very light in colour. The reason why Caucasian hair is so different is because, over many hundreds of years, the nations in Europe have been populated by people from many other countries.

ACTIVITY

Look at the table for some examples and see where you think your own type may have originated from.

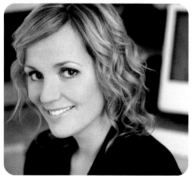

Caucasian type hair

DR JOHN GRAY

IT'S A FACT!

Asian hair grows more quickly than African and Caucasian type hair.

If your hair is ...	It is likely to have originated from ...
Straight and pale blonde	Scandinavia – the countries of Norway, Sweden and Finland.

If your hair is …	It is likely to have originated from …
Dark and straight	Italy and other southern European countries such as Greece.
Red and wavy	Celts from Scotland and Ireland.
Dark, very curly or frizzy	African countries.

IT'S A FACT!

The natural oil of the hair and skin is called sebum. The gland that produces the sebum is called the **sebaceous gland**.

Each hair type varies in shape. If you cut each type of hair in half across the widest part, the cross-section would look like this:

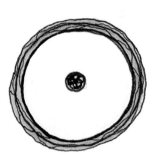

Cross-section of Asian hair

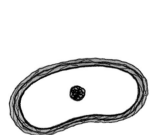

Cross-section of African-type hair   Cross-section of Caucasian hair

WEB LINK

See how the diameter of a hair can vary. Follow the instructions on this web link and change the diameter of a circle. http://www.mathopenref.com/diameter.html

HABIA

Hair texture

Hair texture is the diameter of a single strand of hair. The diameter is the measurement of the widest part of the hair across the centre.

Hair texture can be:

- Fine.
- Medium.
- Coarse.

If you have fine hair, the diameter of your hair will be smaller than that of someone who has coarse hair.

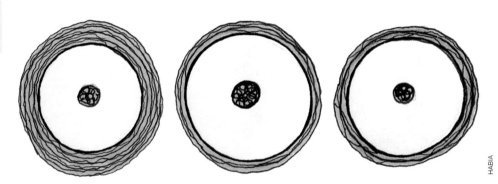

Cross-sections of hair showing increasing number of cuticle layers

HABIA

Hair condition

The condition of your hair can be:

- Dry.
- Oily.
- Normal.

If you have dry hair it can mean the gland that produces the natural oil of the hair is not producing enough oil. If you have oily hair, the gland can be producing too much oil.

Hair can also be dry because it has been damaged. The damage can happen for a number of different reasons. For example you may:

- Cause chemical damage by using too many chemicals such as colour and relaxer.
- Cause chemical damage by using your hair straighteners too much and at too high a temperature.
- Cause environmental damage by exposing the hair to too much sunlight.

ACTIVITY

Compare the diameter of hair in your class. Investigate who has the finest hair and who has the coarsest.

SIGNPOST PLTS

Teamworker
Creative thinker
Reflective learner

SIGNPOST PSD

Healthy living
When you learn about healthy living, you will see how having a poor diet can affect more than your body weight. Read about the foods you need to liven up your dull hair and try out the quiz on the web link to see if you know which foods are good for you.
http://www.nhs.uk/LiveWell/ Goodfood/Pages/ Goodfoodhome.aspx

ACTIVITY

Complete the following activity sheet to find the condition of your hair.

How often do you shampoo your hair?

a I have to shampoo my hair every day.

b I have to shampoo my hair every 3–5 days.

c I only need to shampoo my hair once each week.

What does your hair look like?

a My hair looks lifeless if I do not shampoo it every day.

b My hair is shiny.

c My hair looks dull.

What does your scalp look like?

a I have sticky scales on my scalp.

b I have no scales on my scalp.

c I have flaky skin on my scalp.

Results

Mainly **a** You have oily hair.

Mainly **b** You have normal hair.

Mainly **c** You have dry hair.

www

WEB LINK

How good is your diet? Find out by doing this quiz: **http://www.nhs.uk//Tools/Pages/HealthyEating.aspx**

Hair density

Hair density means the numbers of hairs you have on your head.

Some people have very fine hair that is also **sparse**. This means that they do not have a great number of hairs on their head. You may even be able to see the scalp through their hair. Other people have a lot of hair and this is known as **abundant** hair. This means that they have a great number of hairs on their head.

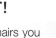

IT'S A FACT!

The number of hairs you have on your head can vary from an average of 100 000 up to 140 000.

Hair length

Hair can be long or short. It can be layered, or the hair can be all the same length. The length of hair will determine the type of hairstyle you can have. Your hair may be too long for a chosen hairstyle, or you may have to grow your hair before you can achieve the hairstyle of your dreams.

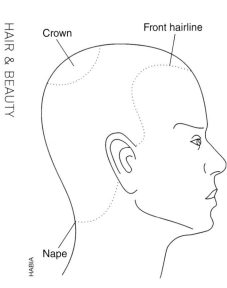

Head showing different areas for hair growth patterns

Hair growth patterns

Hair also grows in different directions on the head. You notice these **hair growth patterns** at the front hairline, the nape of the neck and the crown area. Sometimes you may have a problem hair growth pattern, which means that the hair will not lie in the way you would like it to.

Name of hair growth pattern	Where you find it	What it looks like
Cow lick	Front hairline	Hair grows in an upward direction at the front hairline.
Widow's peak	Front hairline	Hair grows towards the centre at the front hairline.
Double crown	Top of the head	Hair grows in a circular direction at the crown area in two separate places.

Name of hair growth pattern	Where you find it	What it looks like
Nape whorls	Nape of the neck	Hair grows in different directions at the nape of the neck.

HABIA

ACTIVITY

Work with a partner and find the different hair growth patterns you both have. Record the hair growth patterns on the activity sheet.

Front hairline

Do you have?

- Cow lick. ☐
- Widow's peak. ☐
- Neither of these. ☐

Crown

Do you have?

- A single crown. ☐
- A double crown. ☐

Nape

Which direction does the hair at the nape of your neck grow?

- Hair that grows from the right side to the left. ☐
- Hair that grows from the left side to the right. ☐
- Hair that grow away from the centre towards the front. ☐
- Hair that grows into the centre. ☐
- None of these. ☐

SIGNPOST
PLTS

Teamworker
Creative thinker
Independent enquirer

ACTIVITY

Find out which hair growth patterns other members of your class have found. Take photographs of the more unusual hair growth patterns, label them and place them on a poster.

WHAT'S NEXT?

When you progress to Level 1 or Level 2 hairdressing or barbering course you will learn how to analyze the hair growth patterns and the condition of the hair and scalp of clients before you can carry out hairdressing services.

Hair growth cycle

As well as hair growing in different directions on the head, it also grows for a certain length of time. There are times when the hair will fall out and a new hair will grow. This is known as the **hair growth cycle**.

Have you noticed that some people are able to grow their hair really long, while others can't seem to gain any length at all? There are three different stages for

WHAT'S NEXT?

When you progress to Level 2 hair growth cycle you will learn about the different stages of hair growth. They are called **anagen**, **catagen** and **telogen**.

WWW

WEB LINK

Some people are able to grow their hair really long. Look at the length of hair of Xie Qiuping from China: **http://www.guinness worldrecords.com/records/ human_body/extreme_ bodies/default.aspx**

hair growth. The length that your hair grows to is decided by how long each stage lasts. The stage where the hair actively grows varies from one person to another. For some people the active growing stage only lasts for about one year. But some people have an active growing stage that lasts for more than seven years.

Head and face shapes

Apart from identical twins, we all look very different. One reason for this is the shape of our heads and faces. It is the structure of the bones that make the face and head the shape it is.

Head shapes

Everyone has a different head shape. If you have long hair, or very abundant hair, you may not be able to see the shape of your head very well. But if you have very short hair you will be able to see your head shape.

Head shapes

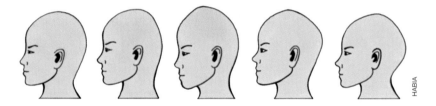

HABIA

Face shapes

The shape of the face can be:

- Oval.
- Round.
- Square.
- Rectangular.
- Long.
- Heart or triangular.
- Pear.
- Diamond.

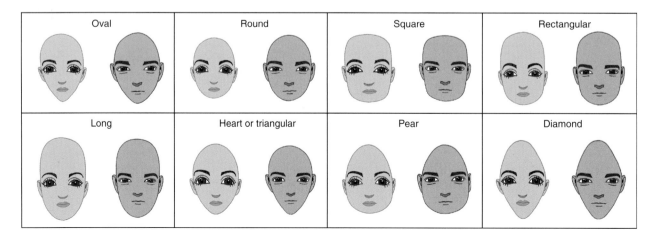

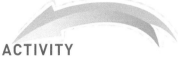

ACTIVITY

Take all the hair away from your face, then work with a partner (or look in a mirror), and identify the shape of your face. Use the information in the table below and the measurements from the diagram to help you.

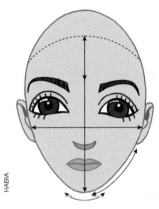

HABIA

Measurements of facial shape

Identify the length of your face and shape of your jaw, chin and forehead		A, B or C?
1 Length of your face		
Is the length of your face much longer than the width?	A	
Is the length of your face the same as the width?	B	
Is the length of your face slightly longer than the width?	C	
2 Jaw line shape		
Is the shape of your jaw line angular?	A	
Is the shape of your jaw line curved?	B	
Is the width of your jaw line wider than your forehead?	C	
3 Chin shape		
Does your chin have a pointed shape?	A	
Does your chin have a curved shape?	B	
4 Forehead		
Is the shape of your hairline angular?	A	

SIGNPOST
PLTS

Reflective learner
Creative thinker

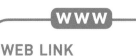

Identify the length of your face and shape of your jaw, chin and forehead		A, B or C?
Is the shape of your hairline round?	B	
Is the width of your hairline narrower than your jaw line?	C	
		Write your results here 1 2 3 4

What is your facial shape? Find your answer results below, but remember there will be slight differences that decide the actual shape of the face.

Results

ABBB = your face shape is oblong

AABA = your face shape is rectangular

ABAC = your face shape is diamond

BABA = your face shape is square

BBBB = your face shape is round

CBBB = your face shape is oval

CAAA = your face shape is triangular

CCBB = your face shape is pear

Finding a hairstyle to suit the shape of your face

To look your best, you should have a hairstyle that suits the shape of your face. For example, if you have a narrow forehead then a heavy fringe may not suit you. If you have a very long face then a hairstyle that is flat at the sides with height at the top may not suit you.

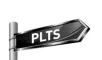

How to prepare for hair care services

Hair care is all about keeping your hair and scalp in good condition. To do this you have to use the correct tools and equipment and know how to shampoo and condition the hair. You must carry out shampoo and conditioning services safely and hygienically. You must prevent harm to yourself and to your client.

Tools and equipment for hair care services

The tools and equipment you need to care for the hair are:

- Combs.
- Hair brushes.
- Sectioning clips.

Combs

A variety of combs will be used for hair care. The combs must be made of materials that will not damage the hair or scalp.

Combs are used to remove tangles from the hair and to section and prepare the hair during treatments and services. You must make sure that you use the correct comb for the task you are completing. You can find details about combs in Chapter 8, 'The art of dressing and styling hair'.

Hairbrushes

Hairbrushes are used to style the hair. You will need to have a variety of different types of brush for different purposes. Some brushes will be used during blow drying to add curl and volume to hair, others will be used to blend and style hair after setting. You can find details about hair brushes in Chapter 8, 'The art of dressing and styling hair'.

Sectioning clips

Sectioning the hair will help you to work neatly. Although you may think that it takes time to section the hair, you will be able to work more quickly as the hair will be tidy. You can find details about sectioning clips in Chapter 8, 'The art of dressing and styling hair'.

Shampooing and conditioning the hair

If you want to have a hairstyle that looks amazing, the starting point has to be hair that is clean and in good condition.

When you shampoo and condition hair you must be able to:

- Prepare for the shampooing and conditioning service following safe and hygienic practices.
- Shampoo, condition and towel dry the hair.

WHAT'S NEXT?

When you progress to Level 2 hairdressing or barbering course you will learn how to analyze the shape of the face so that you can advise clients about hairstyles that will suit them.

TOP TIP

Do not use combs that are made of metal or nylon. Metal combs will tear the hair and create damage. Nylon combs will create static electricity in the hair, making it difficult to manage.

TOP TIP

When you are blow drying hair you section the hair not being dried out of the way. Then you can clearly see the section you are drying. This also stops the wet hair and the dry hair mixing together.

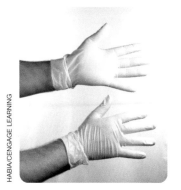

HABIA/CENGAGE LEARNING

Gloved hands

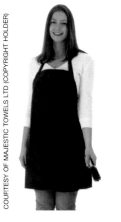

COURTESY OF MAJESTIC TOWELS LTD (COPYRIGHT HOLDER)

Wearing an apron will protect your clothes from splashes

TOP TIP

When you have completed shampoo and conditioning services, wipe the basin, taps and work area so it looks clean for the next client.

IT'S A FACT!

If you are an apprentice or salon junior, you will have to get the tools and equipment ready for more senior members of staff.

Preparing for the shampoo and conditioning service

You must always be prepared when you are working with clients or helping others who are working with clients. When you prepare for the shampoo and conditioning service you have to:

- Prepare yourself.
- Prepare the tools, equipment and protective clothing.
- Prepare the client.

Prepare yourself Before you carry out a shampooing and conditioning service you must protect yourself with personal protective equipment (PPE). You can read more about personal protective equipment in Chapter 9, 'Safe and hygienic working practices'. The personal protective equipment you need for conditioning treatments comprises:

- Apron to keep your clothes clean and to protect you from splashes from the conditioning lotions.
- Gloves to protect your hands and prevent contact dermatitis.

After services such as shampooing hair you must carefully dry your hands. Then apply a good hand cream to moisturize and protect them.

Prepare the tools, equipment and protective clothing You must be prepared and organized for the hair care treatments and services. This is so that work can be carried out safely and efficiently both by you and by other members of staff. To make sure that you are prepared you must collect all the tools and equipment you are going to need before the client service begins. The tools must be sterilized for each new client. The protective clothing must be fresh and clean for each client. You must check that the basin area where the shampoo services are taking place is clean and tidy and free from hair.

The tools and equipment you need for shampooing and conditioning are:

- Combs.
- Brushes.
- Sectioning clips.

The protective clothing you need to prepare for the client is:

- Gown.
- Waterproof shampoo cape.
- Towels.

Prepare the client Before the client's hair is shampooed and conditioned, the hair must be analyzed so that you know which products should be used. You need to know:

- The condition of the client's hair and scalp – so you can use the correct products.
- The length of the client's hair so you can use the correct massage techniques.

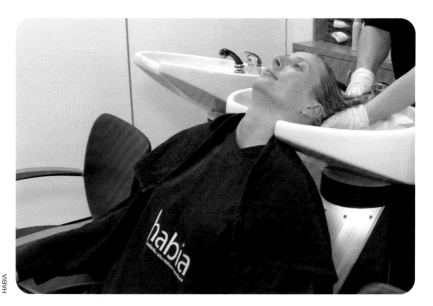

Client prepared for shampooing and conditioning

WHAT'S NEXT?

When you progress to Level 2 hairdressing or barbering you will have to make your own decisions about which shampooing and conditioning products to use for clients, based on the hair analysis you have carried out.

Shampoo, condition and towel dry the hair

The purpose of shampooing is to clean the hair by removing the dirt, hair products and the dead skin scales from the scalp. The purpose of a conditioning service is to improve or maintain the overall condition of the hair.

Before you can begin the shampoo and conditioning service you have to know which products to use.

Shampoo and conditioning products

There are so many products available that it can become quite confusing. But, if you look carefully, you will see that the products are grouped so you can choose one from a group that is suitable for your client. There will be products for different hair and scalp conditions, for different hair types and hair textures.

During the hair and scalp analysis you will find out:

- The hair type of your client.
- The hair texture of your client.
- The condition of the hair and scalp.

Shampoos and conditioning products for different hair types

Hair type refers to the amount of curl in the hair. Some shampoos and conditioners are designed for use on very curly or frizzy hair. These shampoos will have special ingredients which smooth and coat the cuticle layer to make the hair easier to comb. They will also make the hair shine. Shampoos and conditioners for very straight hair are designed to enhance the glossy appearance that it is possible to achieve with flat, straight hair.

Shampoos and conditioning products for different hair textures

Hair texture refers to the diameter of a single strand of hair. Very fine hair can be made to look and feel thicker by the special ingredients in some shampoos and conditioners. The ingredients will coat the hair shaft and make the hair feel thicker. Shampoos for very coarse hair will have extra conditioning ingredients to make the coarse hair feel softer and silkier.

Shampoos and conditioning products for different hair and scalp conditions

You need to know if your client's hair is dry, oily or normal, and if the scalp is dry, oily or dandruff affected before you can choose a suitable shampoo or conditioner.

Shampoo

Hair/scalp type	Description	Recommended product
Normal hair	The hair is neither too dry nor too oily. It will look shiny and healthy and be in good condition.	Use herbal shampoos such as those that contain rosemary or soya and frequent wash mild shampoos.
Dry hair	The hair may look dull and feel coarse and dry. It may not be very shiny.	Use shampoos with additional oily additives, such as those that contain jojoba, coconut or almond.
Dry scalp	The scalp may feel and look tight. There may be some dry skin scales on the scalp. The scalp may feel itchy.	Use products with additives such as juniper or oil-based shampoos containing almond, coconut or olive oil to moisturize and soothe the scalp.
Greasy hair/scalp	The hair may look lank and dull. It will become oily very quickly and need to be washed frequently.	Use camomile shampoos that contain citric acid (lemon, lime, etc.) or mild, frequent use shampoos.
Dandruff affected	The scalp will have loose, dry, white scales which fall onto the shoulders of the client. The scalp may feel itchy.	Use special treatment shampoos for dandruff affected hair to sooth the itchy scalp.

WHAT'S NEXT?

When you progress to Level 2 hairdressing or barbering you will learn more about the chemicals and ingredients found in shampoos. For example, in shampoo for dandruff affected hair you will find **zinc pyrithione** or **selenium sulphide**.

Conditioner

There are two different types of conditioner:

- Surface conditioners.
- Penetrating or treatment conditioners.

Surface conditioners

Surface conditioners work by coating the outside layer of the hair known as the cuticle. Surface conditioners are applied after the shampoo. When you have applied conditioner, the hair is easier to comb. Once you have dried the hair, the cuticle scales lay flat and the hair will look shinier.

You should use a surface conditioner on the following hair conditions:

- Dry.
- Normal.
- Chemically treated.
- Oily hair.

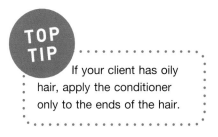

Penetrating or treatment conditioners

You can use a penetrating or treatment conditioner if your client's hair is in very poor condition. Sometimes hair is naturally very dry because the sebaceous glands that produce the natural oil, sebum, are under-productive. Or perhaps the hair may have been damaged by chemicals, heat or the environment.

A penetrating or treatment conditioner is applied to hair that has been shampooed, and then heat is added. The added heat opens the cuticle layer, allowing the conditioner to enter the hair shaft. You can use a variety of electrical equipment to add heat during a conditioning treatment.

The electrical equipment used for penetrating conditioners includes:

- Steamer.
- Accelerator.
- Infrared heater.

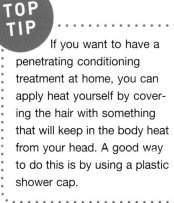

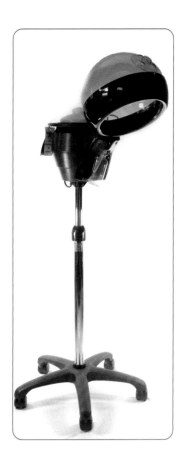

Steamers and accelerators are used to open the cuticle during a penetrating conditioning treatment

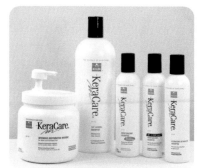

Shampoo and conditioning products for African type hair by Avlon

Conditioner types

● Dry hair and scalp: Use conditioners that contain moisturizers, lanolin or vegetable oils.

● Damaged hair: Use a penetrating conditioner that contains moisturizers or proteins which will temporarily repair internal damage to the cortex.

Images of shampoo and conditioning products

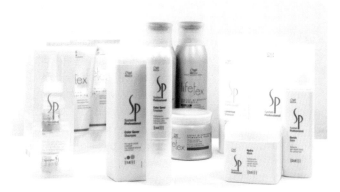

Shampoo and conditioning products by Wella

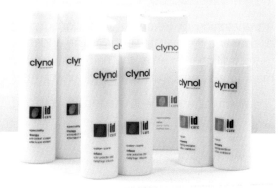

Shampoo and conditioning products by Clynol

SIGNPOST
PLTS

Independent enquirer
Creative thinker

ACTIVITY

Investigate the full range of shampooing and conditioning products by looking on the manufacturer's websites. Useful links are **www.clynol.com www.loreal.co.uk**, **www2.wella.co.uk** and **www.avlon.com**

When you look at the websites you will find information about each product. Work with a partner and choose a range of products that would be good for their hair type, texture and condition. When you have chosen the products make a short presentation to your partner to explain how each product will improve the condition of their hair.

SIGNPOST
FUNCTIONAL
SKILL

English

When you investigate and read about the different products that you would use for your partner, you will:

E3 understand the main point of texts and obtain specific information

L1 identify the main points and ideas and they are presented in different texts.

ACTIVITY

When you get the chance to use different types of shampoo and conditioning product, compare them. You might find that you like some better than others. When you have used them, complete the table below.

Product	Why I liked this product	Results
Write the manufacturer's name and the brand name of the product that you used in this column.	State why you liked the product – for example, did you like the smell, how it felt, how it was packaged, how it looked?	Write down the results achieved from using the product. For example, did the products leave the hair in good condition; perhaps the shampoo lathered well or left the hair tangle free? Perhaps the product was easy to rinse from the hair.

Scalp massage used for shampooing and conditioning

One of the best things about having your hair shampooed and conditioned in a professional salon is the scalp massage.

There are different massage movements and when you are shampooing your client you must use the correct movements to ensure that the massage is comfortable.

SIGNPOST
PLTS

Independent enquirer
Creative thinker
Reflective learner

TOP TIP

When carrying out the scalp massage techniques; use the pads of your fingers and not the tips. Ensure that your nails are not too long.

Massage	Used for	Massage movement	Purpose
Effleurage.	Shampooing and conditioning.	Smooth, flowing, stroking action. Effleurage movement	• Spreads the shampooing and conditioning products. • Cleanses the lengths of long hair during the shampoo process. The stroking movement ensures that the long hair does not tangle. • Ensures that conditioner is spread to the lengths and ends of long hair.

IT'S A FACT!

The petrissage movement is similar to rotary, with a very slight difference. During the rotary movement, the *fingers move across the surface of the scalp*. But, during the petrissage movement, the *fingers move the scalp over the bones of the head*, so a little more pressure is required. The petrissage movement is much slower than the rotary movement.

TOP TIP
Practice the shampoo and conditioning massage movements on your arm so you can see the different amount of pressure that is required.

TOP TIP
You must ensure that you remove all products that have been used for shampooing and conditioning. If you do not, the hair will look lank and dull.

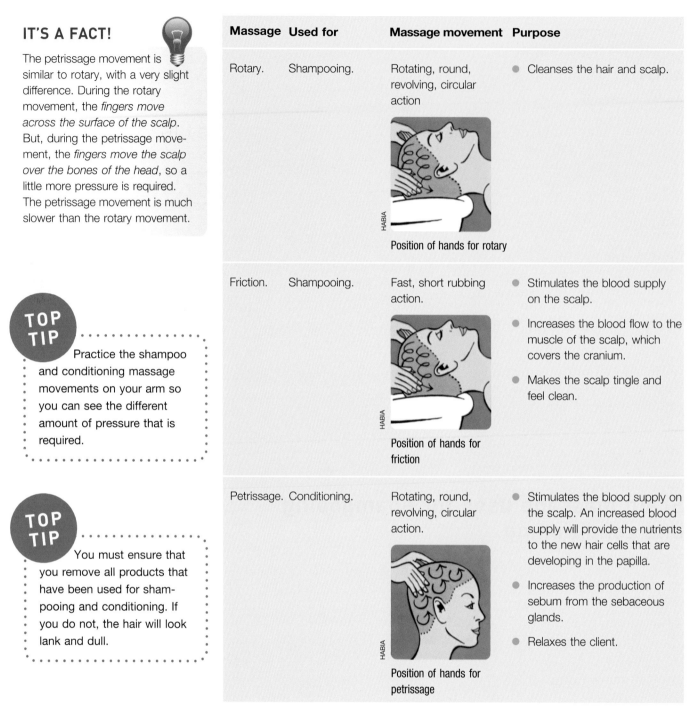

Massage	Used for	Massage movement	Purpose
Rotary.	Shampooing.	Rotating, round, revolving, circular action	• Cleanses the hair and scalp.
Friction.	Shampooing.	Fast, short rubbing action.	• Stimulates the blood supply on the scalp. • Increases the blood flow to the muscle of the scalp, which covers the cranium. • Makes the scalp tingle and feel clean.
Petrissage.	Conditioning.	Rotating, round, revolving, circular action.	• Stimulates the blood supply on the scalp. An increased blood supply will provide the nutrients to the new hair cells that are developing in the papilla. • Increases the production of sebum from the sebaceous glands. • Relaxes the client.

Position of hands for rotary

Position of hands for friction

Position of hands for petrissage

At the end of shampooing and conditioning the hair and scalp, the hair should be gently towel dried to remove excess moisture prior to hairstyling.

Towel drying the hair

When you have completed a shampoo or condition service or treatment the client has to move from the basin back to the styling station. To ensure that the client is comfortable, and does not get wet, you need to wrap the hair in a clean towel. Before removing the towel you can very gently squeeze out excess water before combing the hair with a wide-toothed comb.

Step-by-step methods for shampooing hair

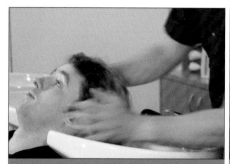

1 The client is gowned for a shampoo and the head is positioned for client comfort and to ensure a water tight seal at the basin. Check that the towel is not trapped between the neck and the basin.

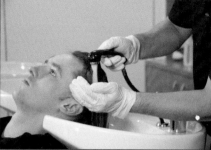

2 Protective gloves are worn and the temperature of the water is tested to ensure client comfort. The hair is evenly wet prior to the application of the shampoo. Note how the hand is cupped near the ear to prevent water running onto the client's face.

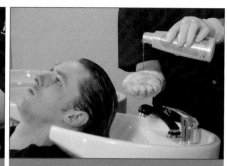

3 Shampoo is poured into the palm of the hand prior to applying to the scalp.

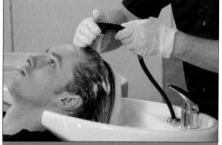

4 *Effleurage* is used to spread the shampoo evenly through the hair and then the scalp is cleansed using rotary and *friction* techniques. The hair is shampooed twice.

5 Shampoo is rinsed from the hair ensuring the scalp and hair are free from product.

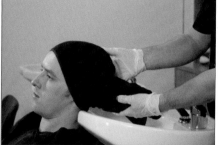

6 A towel is wrapped around the head at the end of the shampoo treatment.

TOP TIP

When you comb the hair after a shampoo and conditioning treatment to remove tangles, always use a wide-toothed comb. Start at the points of the hair and work towards the roots to prevent damage.

TOP TIP

Rinse all the shampoo and conditioning products from the hair. If you do not, the hair will look lank and dull.

Step-by-step methods for conditioning hair with a penetrating conditioner

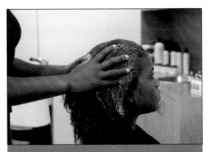

1 The conditioning product is placed into a small bowl.

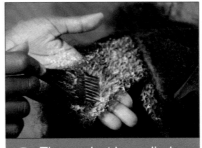

2 The product is applied to the hair using a tinting brush.

3 An *effleurage* massage technique is used to spread the conditioning product evenly through the lengths of the hair.

TOP TIP

When combing conditioner through the hair lengths always use a wide-toothed comb.

ACTIVITY

When you are in the training salon or in your work placement, work with a partner to shampoo and condition each other's hair. When you do this for the first time, you should ask your partner for feedback about the pressure you are using for the massage techniques. Make sure that you have massaged all areas of the scalp. Check that the pressure is comfortable and relaxing. When you have finished the service, write down your experiences. Have a photograph taken of yourself when carrying out the shampoo service. How professional do you look?

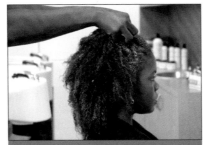

4 The hair is lifted to ensure the finger tips can touch the scalp. The massage is carried out using a *petrissage* massage.

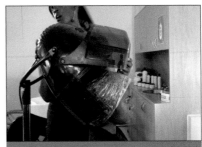

5 To retain the body heat a plastic head cap is placed over the scalp. A hair dryer is used to add additional heat. The additional heat will allow the cuticle scale to lift, and for the product to enter under the cuticle scales. At the end of the treatment, the conditioner is rinsed from the hair ensuring the product is removed from the scalp and hair.

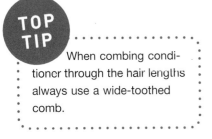

English

When you write about your shampooing and conditioning hair experience, you will:

E3   write text logically and clearly; remember to check your work for accuracy

L1   write text giving your opinions and ideas in a logical sequence; check that you have used correct grammar, punctuation and spelling.

SIGNPOST FUNCTIONAL SKILL

SIGNPOST PLTS

Reflective learner
Teamworker

What you have learnt

The basic structure of the hair

- The hair is made of keratin.
- The hair is made of three sections.
- The hair has many appendages found in the dermis of the skin.

How to analyze your hair

- Hair type means how curly or straight your hair is.
- Hair texture is the diameter of a single strand of hair.
- Hair condition means how dry or oily your hair is.
- Hair length means how long or short your hair is.

How hair grows

- There are different patterns of hair growth found at the nape, the crown and the front hairline.
- The three different stages of hair growth are anagen, catagen and telogen.

Head and face shapes

- There are different head and face shapes which are formed by the bones of the head and face.

How to prepare for hair care services

- How to use and prepare the correct combs, brushes and sectioning clips.
- How to prepare yourself and client for shampooing and conditioning services.

Shampooing and conditioning the hair

- There are different types of shampoo and conditioner for a range of hair and scalp conditions.
- The massage movements used for shampooing and conditioning.
- How to safely carry out the shampooing and conditioning services.

ASSESSMENT ACTIVITIES

Activity 1 E3 – L1

These are multiple choice questions. Read through each question carefully. When you have finished, tick the correct answer.

1 Hair is made from a:

    a. Protein.   c. Mineral.

    b. Vitamin.   d. Fat.

2 The number of layers that can be found in hair is:

    a. 1   c. 5

    b. 3   d. 7

3 The outside layer of the hair is called the:

    a. Medulla.

    b. Cortex.

    c. Keratin.

    d. Cuticle.

4 The tube-like structure that holds the hair in place is called the:

    a. Follicle.

    b. Arrector pili muscle.

    c. Papilla.

    d. Sebaceous gland.

5 Hair type means:

    a. How weak or strong the hair is.

    b. How dry or oily the hair is.

    c. How curly or straight the hair is.

    d. How coarse or fine the hair is.

6 A widow's peak is found at:

    a. Side of the head.   c. Nape.

    b. Front hairline.   d. Crown.

7 A comb used for removing tangles in hair should:

    a. Have wide teeth.

    b. Have narrow teeth.

    c. Be made from plastic.

    d. Be made from metal.

8 When combing tangles from hair:

    a. Start at the front.

    b. Start at the roots.

    c. Start at the back.

    d. Start at the ends.

9 When shampooing your client's hair you must wear:

    a. A uniform.   c. A gown.

    b. Protective gloves.   d. Flat shoes.

10 A massage only used for shampooing is:

    a. Petrissage.   c. Effleurage.

    b. Rotary.   d. Gentle.

Activity 2 E1 – L1

Place the sentences below into the correct order for shampooing a client:

Wet the hair.

Wrap the hair in a towel.

Gown the client.

Rinse the hair.

Put on protective gloves.

Place a waterproof cape around the shoulders of the client.

Shampoo the hair.

Analyze the hair to determine which shampoo to use.

Check the temperature of the water.

Place a towel around the shoulders of the client.

1	
2	
3	
4	
5	
6	
7	
8	
9	
10	

Activity 3 E3 – L1

Work with a partner or split into two teams. Choose a letter and answer the question. When you have answered the question correctly, mark off your square. See who can correctly answer the questions to complete a straight or diagonal line across the grid. You can block the way of your partner or other team to stop them winning!

C	T	O	R	T
W	D	T	S	S
A	E	C	P	R
M	F	W	G	P
P	S	A	D	E

C	Which C is the inner layer of hair? _____
W	Which W is a hair growth pattern found at the nape of the neck? _____
A	Which A is the type of hair that is very curly? _____
M	Which M is the section of hair that is sometimes missing? _____
P	Which P is the place where the new hair cells are produced? _____
T	Which T is the name that tells you how curly or straight your hair is? _____
D	Which D tells you how many hairs you have on your head? _____
E	Which E is also known as Caucasian hair? _____
F	Which F is a hair texture? _____

S	Which S is the name for the natural oil of the hair and skin? _____
O	Which O is a name given to the condition of hair? _____
T	Which T is a face shape? _____
C	Which C is a tool that you use for hair care? _____
W	Which W is the type of comb teeth that you use when removing tangles from hair? _____
A	Which A is a comb that can be used on very tightly curled hair? _____
R	Which R is a brush used during blow drying? _____
S	Which S is the name of the clips that keeps the hair neat during blow drying? _____
P	What is the P that you have to be when shampooing the hair of a client? _____
G	Which G will protect your hands during shampooing and conditioning services? _____
D	Which D is the name of a condition that can affect the skin of hands? _____
T	What T is wrapped around the client's head when you have completed the shampoo? _____
S	Which S can be used to open the cuticle of the hair during conditioning treatments? _____
R	Which R is the name of a shampoo massage? _____
P	Which P is the name of a conditioning massage? _____
E	What is the E that you can use for both shampooing and conditioning massages? _____

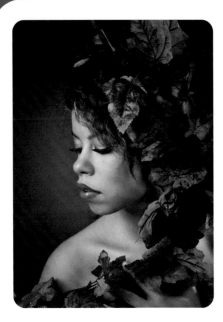

8

The art of styling and dressing hair

"I was the first person to have a punk rock hairstyle.

VIVIENNE WESTWOOD, FASHION DESIGNER

In this chapter you are going to learn about:

- The science behind hair styling.
- The factors that influence the choice of hair styles.
- The tools, products and equipment you will use for plaiting, twisting, styling and dressing hair.
- How to prepare for plaiting, twisting, styling and dressing hair.
- The basic techniques for plaiting, twisting, styling and dressing hair.

Introduction

The way you style and dress your hair can say a great deal about you. Your hairstyle can be a clue to who you are. Some people like to keep their hair covered for religious or cultural reasons. Others like to have theirs on show. You can style your hair in ways to reflect your own personality. On special occasions your hairstyle is as important as the clothes you are wearing. In this chapter you are going to learn about styling the hair of men and women and how to plait and twist hair to create some amazing looks.

The science behind hair styling

Have you noticed that when you style your hair, the style looks nice for a short time and then, especially if your hair gets damp, the style just disappears – and you are left with the hair style you started with!

And, if your hair is naturally curly, have you noticed that when your hair is wet, it can look straight, but then as it dries it begins to curl up into its natural curl?

One reason why your hairstyle reverts to its natural position and why hair looks different when wet than dry is because the hair has properties of **elasticity**. Hair will not stretch like an elastic band, but it does stretch a little, and if it is in good condition, it will go back to its natural length. You can test the amount of elasticity in your hair by carrying out an elasticity test. You can find out more about carrying out an elasticity test in Chapter 7, 'Introduction to hair care'.

When you style your hair you are making a temporary change in the structure of the hair. Because it is temporary, your hairstyle does not last for ever. The reason you can change the structure of your hair is because of some special bonds in the **cortex** of the hair. You can read more about the cortex in Chapter 7, too. The bonds are special because they hold all the cells of the cortex together. They hold the hair cells together in its natural position. So if your hair is naturally curly, the bonds hold your hair in a curly position. If your hair is straight, the bonds will hold your hair in a naturally straight position.

But the bonds are not rigid, they are flexible. When water or heat is used on the hair, some of the bonds move. They move to the place of the hairstyle you want to create. So if your hair is naturally curly and you straighten your hair with a brush and dryer, or with straighteners, the bonds move to the position that makes your hair look straight. And if your hair is naturally straight, and you curl your hair with hair rollers, heated rollers or curling tongs, the bonds move to the position that makes your hair look curly.

IT'S A FACT!

The change in the hair structure during styling is a temporary change. There are some chemical treatments such as perming and relaxing which permanently change the structure of the hair.

WHAT'S NEXT?

When you progress to a higher level hairdressing qualification you will learn that the names of the bonds in the hair that change are called *hydrogen* bonds and the names of the different stages of change the hair goes through when styling are known as *alpha* and *beta* keratin.

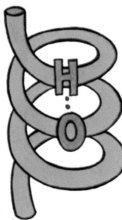
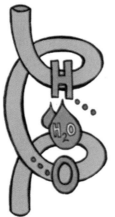
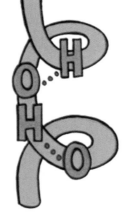

HABIA

The bonds that hold the cells of the hair together are broken by water and heat

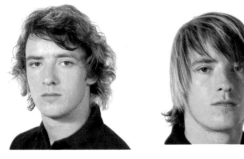

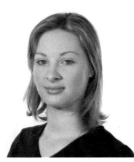

When naturally curly hair is straightened the bonds in the hair reform into a new, temporary position

There is another reason why your hairstyle is only a temporary change to the hair structure. You will find that your hairstyle will last longer on dry, sunny days than it does on foggy days. This is because hair has another special feature. It is able to draw water vapour into itself from the atmosphere. So if you go outside on a humid

When naturally straight hair is curled, the bonds in the hair reform into a new, temporary position day, or are in a steamy bathroom, your new style will not last as long. The damp or humid air taken in by the hair will make the bonds go back to their normal position. The reason hair can draw water vapour into itself is because it is **hygroscopic**.

The factors that influence the choice of hair styles

You need to know which factors will affect the end result of the hair styling service. So before you style, dress, plait or twist hair you must consider the following:

- Hair texture.
- Hair type.
- Hair growth patterns.
- Hair length.
- Hair density.
- Hair elasticity.
- Face shape.
- Head shape.

You can read more about all the factors that influence hairstyling in Chapter 7.

When you carry out a client consultation for styling, dressing, plaiting or twisting hair, ask yourself the following questions.

Hair texture

Is the hair the correct texture for the style you want to achieve? Some hair may be too fine to achieve a 'big hair' result. Other hair may be too coarse for a sleek result.

Hair type

Is the hair too straight or too curly for the style you want to achieve? If hair is very curly and frizzy, you may damage the hair by straightening it too much. If hair is very straight, a curled result may not last very long.

Hair growth patterns

Are there any hair growth patterns that might prevent you from having the hairstyle you want to achieve? For example, if you have a cow lick, you might not be able to have a full fringe as the cow lick will not allow the hair to lie evenly.

Hair length

Is the hair too long or too short for the style you want to achieve? Some clients may have to grow their hair to get their dream look. Others may need to have their hair cut.

Hair density

Is the hair too abundant or too fine for the style you want to achieve? If hair is sparse, you will not be able to achieve a 'big hair' result. If hair is too abundant, it may be difficult to achieve a style that is flat and close to the head.

Hair elasticity

Is the hair in good condition? Hair in poor condition will not curl as well as hair in good condition. This is because hair that is in poor condition will have reduced elasticity. The elasticity will be reduced because some of the bonds that hold the cortex together are missing or damaged.

Face shape

Is the face the best shape for the style you want to achieve? If you have an oval face, then any style will suit you. But if your face is very round, you might want to avoid a heavy fringe that would make the face look even shorter. If your face is oblong, you might want to have a fringe to make the face look more oval.

Head shape

Is the head the best shape for the style you want to achieve? If the head shape is very uneven, you might want to avoid a style that is very close to the head.

ACTIVITY

This two-part activity will let you see how the factors that affect hairstyling can determine if a hairstyle is suitable for you or for a client.

PART 1 Ask a partner to analyze your hair, head and face shape first and then you should analyze the hair, head and face shape of your partner. Only complete parts a–h on the consultation sheet for hair styling for this first activity. If necessary, refer to Chapter 7 for further information about analysing your hair, head and face shape.

When you have completed parts a–h, you can move on to Part 2 of the activity.

PART 2 Look in a hairstyle magazine and choose a new hairstyle for yourself and then work with a partner to choose another hairstyle for them. Then complete parts 1–8 of the consultation sheet to check if the hairstyles are suitable and possible to achieve.

CONSULTATION SHEET FOR HAIR STYLING, DRESSING, PLAITING AND TWISTING HAIR

Head shape
Tick the box that best represents the head shape:

a.

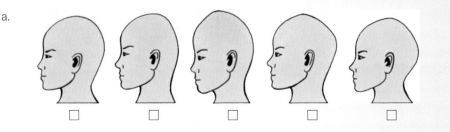

IT'S A FACT!

Hair elasticity is even more important when you are plaiting hair. Excessive tension during plaiting on hair can lead to hair damage. You must always check for signs of **traction alopecia** before plaiting or twisting hair.

IT'S A FACT!

Traction alopecia is caused by excessive tension on hair, leading to hair loss, especially around the hairline. This can happen during plaiting and twisting, or even wearing tight pony tails.

ACTIVITY

Investigate the symptoms of traction alopecia. If you key *traction alopecia* into a search engine you can find lots of images of the condition.

SIGNPOST PLTS

Independent enquirer

WEB LINK

When you carry out part 2 of the activity, look at this website. There are nearly 8,000 hairstyles to choose from. Have a look to see if there are any that you like. http://www.ukhairdressers.com/Style%20Gallery.asp

WEB LINK

Have a look at this web link for a virtual salon to help choose a hairstyle: http://www.ukhairdressers.com/virtual%20salon.asp. You can try out different hairstyles on different shaped faces. You can even change the colour of the hairstyle. On the same website you can upload your own image and try out celebrity hairstyles to see if they will suit you.

SIGNPOST PLTS

Independent enquirer
Creative thinker
Teamworker

1 Will the hairstyle you have chosen be suitable for the head shape and make it appear evenly shaped?   Yes ☐ No ☐

Face shape
Tick the box that best represents the face shape:

b.

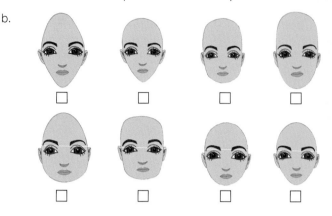

☐   ☐   ☐   ☐

☐   ☐   ☐   ☐

2 Will the hairstyle you have chosen be suitable for the face shape?   Yes ☐ No ☐

Hair growth
Tick the boxes that match the hair growth patterns:

c. ☐ Cow lick ☐ widow's peak ☐ nape whorl ☐ single crown ☐ double crown

3 Is the hairstyle you have chosen possible to achieve with the hair growth patterns?   Yes ☐ No ☐

Hair length
Tick the box(es) that match the hair length:

d. ☐ Short ☐ shoulder length ☐ long ☐ very long ☐ layered ☐ not layered

4 Is the hair the right length for the hairstyle you have chosen?   Yes ☐ No ☐

Hair type
Tick the box that matches the hair type:

e. ☐ Frizzy ☐ very curly ☐ curly ☐ very wavy ☐ wavy ☐ straight

5 Is the hair the correct type to achieve the hairstyle you have chosen?   Yes ☐ No ☐

Hair texture
Tick the box that matches the hair texture:

f. ☐ Very coarse ☐ coarse ☐ medium ☐ fine ☐ very fine

6 Is the hair the correct texture to achieve the hairstyle you have chosen?   Yes ☐ No ☐

Hair elasticity
Tick the box that matches the elasticity of the hair (you will need to do an elasticity test):

g. ☐ Very good elasticity ☐ good elasticity ☐ poor elasticity

7 Is there sufficient elasticity in the hair to achieve and maintain the hairstyle?   Yes ☐ No ☐

Hair density
Tick the box that best matches the density of the hair:

h. ☐ Very abundant ☐ abundant ☐ medium ☐ sparse ☐ very sparse

8 Is the density suitable to achieve the hairstyle you have chosen?   Yes ☐ No ☐

ICT

When you look at a virtual salon on the web link, you will interact with ICT for a given purpose and you will be able to recognize and use interface features. **E1 – L1**

SIGNPOST FUNCTIONAL SKILL

The tools, equipment and products you will use for plaiting, twisting, styling and dressing hair

There is a wide range of tools, equipment and products that you can use for plaiting, twisting, styling and dressing hair.

Combs

You will need a variety of combs to carry out combing and sectioning techniques for plaiting, twisting, styling and dressing on different types and textures of hair. Professional hairdressing combs are made from materials that prevent damage to the hair structure and reduce static electricity. You must ensure that the combs used for clients are sterilized between uses.

	Use	Benefit	Tip
Wide-toothed combs	For combing hair to remove tangles.	The wide teeth are good for coarse, dense hair, or very curly hair.	Always comb hair from the points to the roots to prevent damage.
Wide- and narrow-toothed combs	For combing a variety of hair types and textures.	The wide teeth are good for coarse, dense hair or very curly hair. The fine teeth are good for combing very short hair and backcombing.	Do not use the fine teeth on coarse, curly or frizzy hair. It will be uncomfortable for the client.
Tail combs	For making sections when plaiting, twisting, styling and dressing hair.	The tail of the comb enables you to make clean, neat sections. This means that you will be able to work methodically and efficiently.	Use the point of the tail to make the sections.
Afro pick	For use on very tight, curly or frizzy hair.	The wide teeth make it easier to comb this hair type.	Comb from the outside edges of the hair, into the centre.

COURTESY OF DENMAN INTERNATIONAL LIMITED

Hair brushes

You will need a variety of hair brushes that are suitable for different hair types and textures. The bristles of professional hair brushes are made from materials that are designed to prevent damage to the cuticle and reduce static electricity.

You must ensure that hair brushes used for your clients are sterilized between uses.

	Use	Benefit	Tip
Flat back brushes	For brushing hair during drying and styling.	Removes sectioning marks after setting. Prepares hair for plaiting, twisting, styling and dressing. Removes tangles from hair.	Do not use brushes to remove tangles on wet hair as this would make the hair stretch too much.
Paddle brushes	For brushing hair during drying and styling.	Removes sectioning marks after setting. Removes tangles from hair. Prepares hair for plaiting, twisting, styling and dressing. Massages the scalp.	The cushioned base and gentle bristles means this type of hair brush is good for massaging and stimulating the scalp of dry hair. Do not over use on hair that is naturally oily, as stimulating the scalp will produce more sebum.
Radial brushes	For creating curls in hair when blow drying or for smoothing and straightening curly hair.	Lifts the hair at the roots to create volume.	Use a small radial brush to create tighter curls and a large radial brush for large curls.
Vent brushes	For styling during blow drying.	The open back of the brush allows the air to pass through to quicken the drying time.	Use on short, straight hair to create texture.

Equipment

If you want to create a wide range of hairstyles, you will need a range of equipment.

Some equipment is designed to be used on wet hair, others just for dry hair. All equipment should be made from materials that will not damage the hair.

	Use	Benefit	Tip
Velcro™ rollers	For creating soft curls and movement in hair.	Soft, natural looking curls. Adds volume to hair.	Only use Velcro™ rollers on dry hair. The small teeth on the rollers attach themselves to the hair shaft and will not work on wet hair.
Rollers	For creating curls and movement in hair.	Different size curls can be produced using different sized rollers.	Use large rollers to create big, open curls and small ones for tight curls.
Pin curl clips	For making pin curls in hair.	Make natural looking curls in the hair.	Use small sections when creating the pin curl.
Hair bands, pins and grips	For holding long hair in place.	Keeps a long hair style neatly in place. Hair bands prevent plaits unravelling.	Use dark coloured pins on dark hair and pale coloured pins on light hair to help to disguise them.
Diffuser	Attached to a hand-held dryer.	Dries hair without disturbing natural curl.	Use the dryer speed on a low setting to prevent 'frizzing' curly hair.
Afro pick attachment	Attached to a hand-held dryer.	Straightens very curly hair as it dries.	Keep the dryer on a medium heat to prevent burning the scalp and damaging the hair.
Sectioning clips	To clip hair into sections.	Enables you to work in a logical and methodical way.	When inserting the sectioning clips, open them fully to prevent pulling the hair.

	Use	Benefit	Tip
Back mirror	To enable the client to see the back of the hairstyle.	Ensures the client is happy with the finished result.	Hold the mirror to one side so the image is reflected back into the main mirror.
Trolley	To store tools and equipment.	Keeps tools and equipment safe and tidy.	So you don't have to bend over to reach the trolley, keep it on your right-hand side if you are right handed and vice versa. This will prevent back strain and injury.

Electrical equipment

The range of electrical equipment to style hair is vast. Hair can be dried, curled, straightened, pressed and crimped with specialized equipment. Professional electrical equipment is designed for all-day-long use.

	Use	Benefit	Tip
Hand-held hair dryer	For drying and styling hair.	Portable and easy to use.	Use the different adjustable temperatures and speeds to suit your hair texture and density. Fine hair will need a cooler, slower setting than dense, coarse hair.
Straighteners	For straightening and curling hair.	Can be used to create a variety of effects.	Use moisturizing products to protect the hair from heat damage.
Tongs	For curling hair.	Can be used to create a variety of different sized curls.	Use small barrel tongs to create tight curls and large barrel tongs for soft curls.

	Use	Benefit	Tip
Pressing comb	For smoothing very curly and frizzy hair.	Can be used to smooth and blend unevenly relaxed hair.	Use on the hairline straighten where straighteners cannot reach.
Crimpers	For creating a zigzag or waved appearance to hair.	Can be used to create a variety of looks.	Crimp longer, one-length hair for the best effects. Use just at the roots on short hair to create lift and volume.
Thermal irons	For smooth curls and movement in the hair.	Can be used to create a variety of curl sizes – even on very short hair. Heated in an oven.	Use thermal irons to straighten the regrowth of chemically straightened hair.
Heated rollers	For creating waves, curl and movement.	Can be used on long and short hair to produce a quick result.	Only use on dry hair.
Hood dryer	For drying hair.	The whole head can be dried at the same time.	Check the temperature to ensure client comfort.
Accelerator	To create dry heat.	Can be used to dry hair.	Place the equipment over the whole head to ensure even distribution of heat.

TOP TIP

Always keep yourself up-to-date with your product knowledge. Read manufacturer's instructions on how and when to use a styling product to achieve the best results.

Products for styling hair

When styling hair you will use different products to:

● Protect the hair from heat.

● Strengthen hair with reduced elasticity.

● Extend the life of the finished hairstyle.

● Add moisture.

● Add shine and create texture.

It does not matter what the type, texture or condition of your hair is, you will find a product to help achieve the result you are after.

Different types of styling and finishing product

All product manufacturers will make a range of styling and finishing products for different hair types. Many products can be used in combination with one another to help you provide the result you want to achieve the total look.

Product type	Typical use
Gel	To create a 'wet' look.
Glaze	For additional style hold.
Mousse	For additional style hold.
Wax	To create texture and additional hold.
Serum	To add moisture and increase shine. Helps to create a smoother look on frizzy hair.
Spray	To protect the hair from damp conditions and provide additional hold.

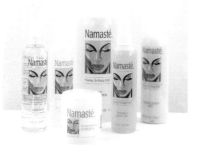

Styling and finishing products for African type hair by Namaste

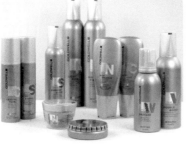

Styling and finishing products by Goldwell

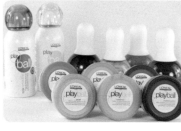

Styling and finishing products by L'Oréal

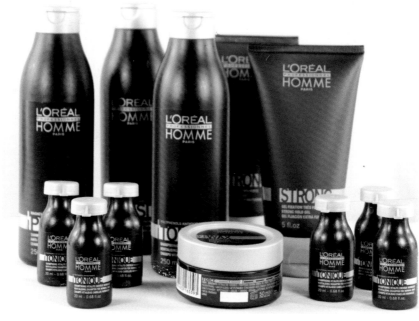

Styling and finishing products for men by L'Oréal

ACTIVITY

Investigate a product range of styling and finishing products. Identify the products that are best used to provide:

- Styling support.
- Added moisture to hair.
- Added strength to hair.
- Added shine to the hair.
- Protection against the environment. For example, from the sun or from swimming.
- Heat protection. For example, from heated styling equipment.
- To increase the life of the hairstyle.

Make an informative leaflet that you could give to clients to tell them about the products.

SIGNPOST PLTS

Independent enquirer
Creative thinker

ICT

When you look at the website to find out information about styling and finishing products, you will interact with ICT for a given purpose and you will be able to recognize and use interface features. **E1 – E3**

SIGNPOST FUNCTIONAL SKILL

English

When you read the information on the website about the styling and finishing products, you will:

E3 and **L1**   read and understand the purpose and context of straightforward texts.

When you write about the styling and finishing products, you will:

E3   plan, draft and organize your writing and write logically and clearly check you grammar, punctuation and spelling

L1   write logically and clearly including an appropriate level of detail. You will use the correct grammar ensuring accurate punctuation and spelling.

SIGNPOST FUNCTIONAL SKILL

WWW

WEB LINK

There are many websites for professional hairdressers which show a range of products for all different hair types and styling applications. Some examples are: **http://www.avlon.com/home.html** or **http://www.loreal professionnel.co.uk/_en/_gb/** or **http://www.clynol.com/products_style_scroll.asp**. Have a look at the Wella site for styling techniques and use of products: **http://www.wella professionals.co.uk/hair dresser/products/styling/high_hair/specials/trend_vision/index.php**

How to prepare for plaiting, twisting, styling and dressing hair

You must always be prepared when you are working with clients or helping others who are working with clients. When you prepare for plaiting, twisting, styling and dressing hair you have to:

- Prepare the tools, equipment and products.
- Prepare the client.

Preparing the tools, equipment and products

You must be prepared and organized for plaiting, twisting, styling and dressing hair. This is so that work can be carried out safely and efficiently. To make sure that you are prepared you must collect all the tools, equipment and products you are going to need.

Preparing the client

Before you can plait, twist, style or dress hair, you must carry out a client consultation. You can read about the factors that affect plaiting, twisting, styling and dressing hair in the first part of this chapter.

You must carry out a consultation with your client before hair styling services

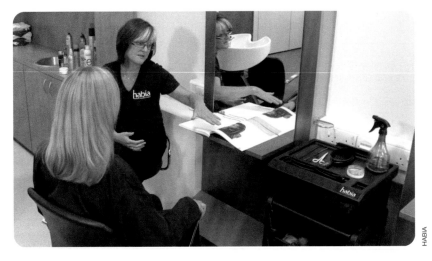

HABIA

TOP TIP If the hair style your client has chosen is not suitable, you must be very tactful when suggesting alternative styles.

TOP TIP The client's hair, whether it is wet or dry, must be carefully combed to remove tangles before plaiting, twisting, styling or dressing hair. Always remove tangles by combing from the points to the roots – never the other way round.

You also need to find out the end result the client would like. Some clients have a very good idea about how they want their hair to look and can describe the style they would like. Other clients may not be able to do this so well. So you may have to use **visual aids**. You can use style books and hairstyle magazines. You might ask the client to bring some pictures with them. Or you may be able to find some examples of styles on the internet. However you show style examples to your client, you must be certain that you can achieve the style they are requesting.

The client's clothes must be protected before you begin plaiting, twisting, styling or dressing the hair. They will require a fresh and clean gown.

The client's hair must be prepared for the plaiting, twisting, styling or dressing service. You may be working on pre-shampooed, wet hair, or you may be working on hair that is shampooed and then dried.

The basic techniques for plaiting, twisting, styling and dressing hair

The number of hairstyles you can create are restricted only by your imagination and the limits found during the client consultation. There are so many hairstyles to choose from. But to create those hairstyles, you will only use a combination of four hairstyling techniques:

- Make hair look curly.

- Make hair look wavy.

- Make hair look straight.

- Plait and twist hair.

Making hair curly

To make hair curly, you can use any of the following methods:

- Set hair in rollers to make a variety of curl shapes.
- Set hair in pin curls to make a variety of curl shapes.
- Set hair in Velcro™ rollers to create soft curls.
- Set hair in heated rollers to create soft curls.
- Curl hair using straighteners to make soft curls.
- Curl hair using tongs to make a variety of different types of curl.
- Blow dry hair using radial hair brushes to make a variety of soft curls and add volume to hair.
- Increase natural curl in hair by using a diffuser attachment with a hand-held dryer.

Making hair wavy

To make hair wavy you can use any of the following methods:

- Loosen and soften existing curls, or create waves in straight hair by setting in rollers.
- Loosen and soften existing curls, or create waves in straight hair by setting in Velcro™ rollers.
- Loosen and soften existing curls, or create waves in straight hair by setting in heated rollers.
- Loosen and soften existing curls, or create waves in straight hair by blow drying with radial brushes.
- Loosen and soften existing curls, or create waves in straight hair using straighteners.
- Wave hair using crimpers to make a variety of different effects from soft waves to frizz.

Making hair straight

With the latest heated electrical equipment and products to protect hair against excessive heat, it is possible temporarily to straighten most hair types with straighteners:

- Straighten by wrapping.
- Straighten by setting hair on very large rollers.
- Straighten using a very large radial brush when blow drying.
- Straighten with electrical equipment.

TOP TIP The prolonged use of straighteners is not recommended as this can lead to hair damage and breakage.

Plaiting and twisting hair

There are many ways in which hair can be plaited and twisted:

- Scalp plaits or twists.
- Fishtail plaits.

- Corn rows.

- Full head or partial head plaits or twists.

- Adding additional hair or materials to plaits or twists

Step-by-step methods for making hair curly and wavy

Creating curls and waves by setting hair in rollers

This technique is used to create longer lasting curls, waves, volume and movement.

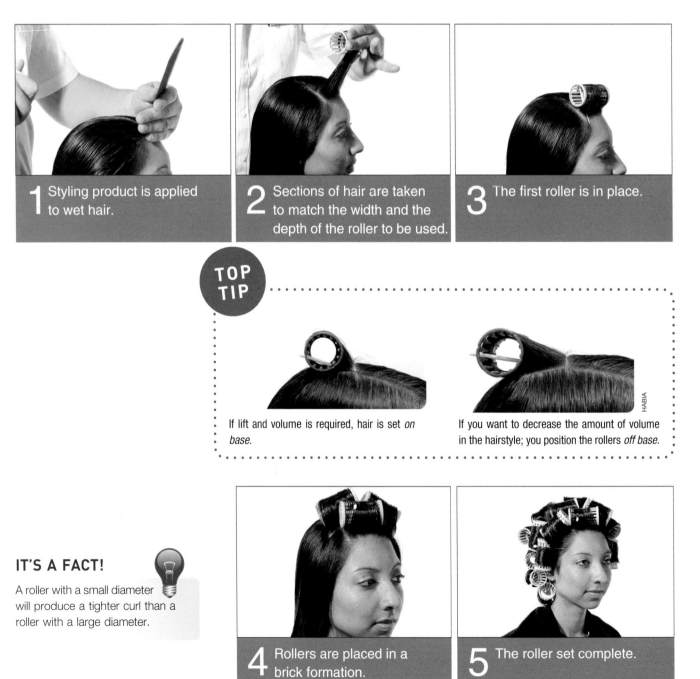

1 Styling product is applied to wet hair.

2 Sections of hair are taken to match the width and the depth of the roller to be used.

3 The first roller is in place.

TOP TIP

If lift and volume is required, hair is set *on base*.

If you want to decrease the amount of volume in the hairstyle; you position the rollers *off base*.

IT'S A FACT!

A roller with a small diameter will produce a tighter curl than a roller with a large diameter.

4 Rollers are placed in a brick formation.

5 The roller set complete.

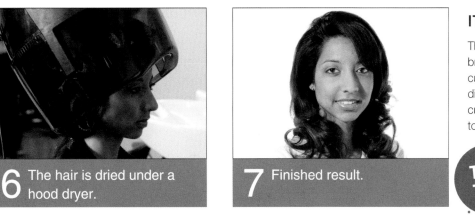

6 The hair is dried under a hood dryer.

7 Finished result.

HABIA AND CENGAGE LEARNING

IT'S A FACT!

The diameter of the radial brush will determine the size of curls you can create. Use a small diameter brush to make tighter curls. Use a large diameter brush to create large curls.

TOP TIP
To prevent burning the client, keep the air from the dryer pointed away from the scalp.

Creating curls and waves by blow drying

A radial brush can be used to create curls, waves, body and movement in hair.

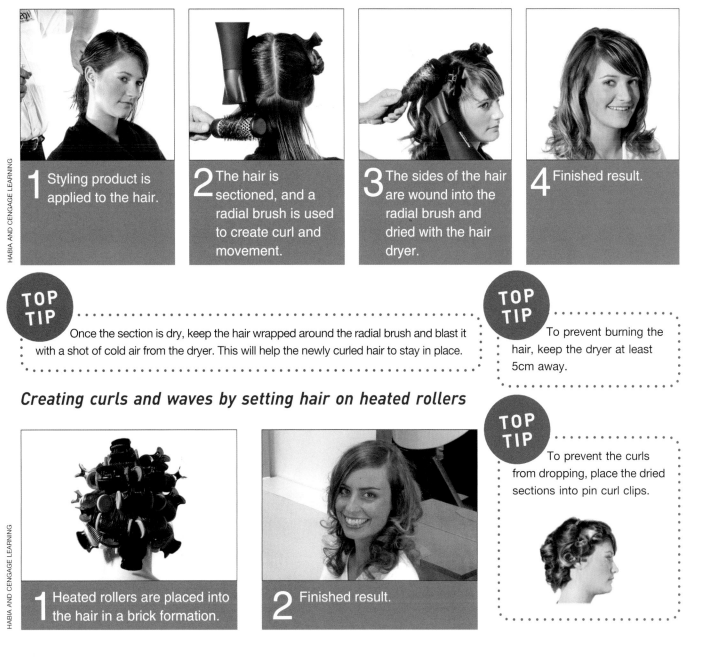

1 Styling product is applied to the hair.

2 The hair is sectioned, and a radial brush is used to create curl and movement.

3 The sides of the hair are wound into the radial brush and dried with the hair dryer.

4 Finished result.

TOP TIP
Once the section is dry, keep the hair wrapped around the radial brush and blast it with a shot of cold air from the dryer. This will help the newly curled hair to stay in place.

TOP TIP
To prevent burning the hair, keep the dryer at least 5cm away.

Creating curls and waves by setting hair on heated rollers

1 Heated rollers are placed into the hair in a brick formation.

2 Finished result.

TOP TIP
To prevent the curls from dropping, place the dried sections into pin curl clips.

HABIA AND CENGAGE LEARNING

Creating curls and waves by setting hair in pin curls

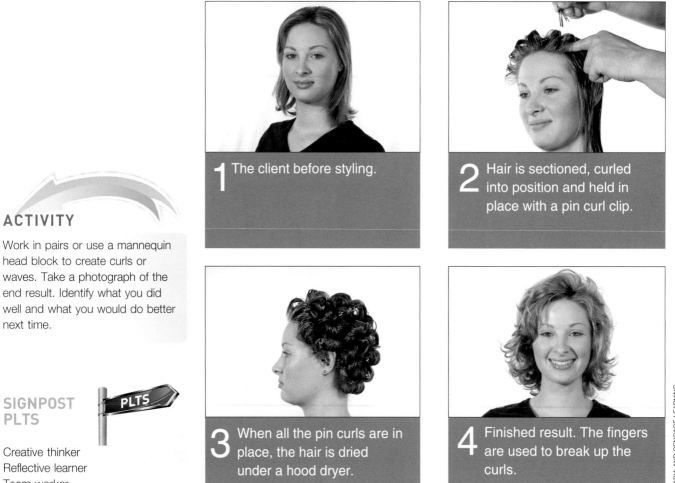

1 The client before styling.

2 Hair is sectioned, curled into position and held in place with a pin curl clip.

3 When all the pin curls are in place, the hair is dried under a hood dryer.

4 Finished result. The fingers are used to break up the curls.

ACTIVITY

Work in pairs or use a mannequin head block to create curls or waves. Take a photograph of the end result. Identify what you did well and what you would do better next time.

SIGNPOST PLTS

Creative thinker
Reflective learner
Team worker
Self manager

Other methods for creating curls and waves in hair

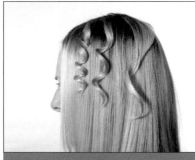

Curling tongs of different sizes will create different sized curls.

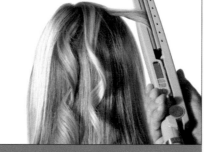

Curls can be created by turning straighteners as they are moved down the hair shaft.

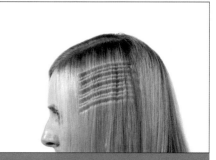

Tight waves can be created by using crimpers.

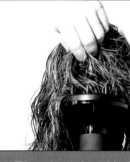

The natural curl in hair can be increased by using a diffuser attachment on a hand-held hair dryer.

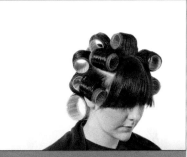

Velcro™ rollers can be used to create soft curls, wave and volume.

Step-by-step methods for making hair straight

With heated electrical equipment and the improvement in products to maintain the condition of hair, it is possible to temporarily straighten most hair types.

TOP TIP ⬤ The prolonged use of straighteners is not recommended as this can lead to hair damage and breakage.

Making hair straight by using a wrapping technique

The wrapping technique is used to smooth hair and uses the shape of the head to create movement.

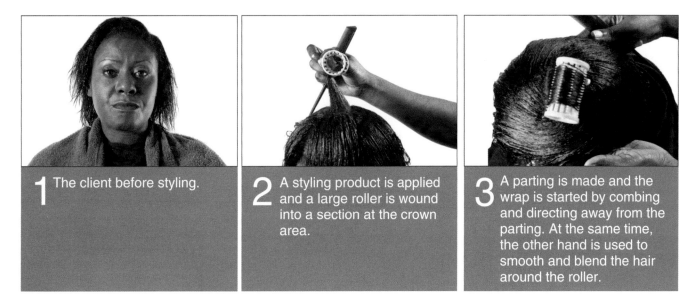

1 The client before styling.

2 A styling product is applied and a large roller is wound into a section at the crown area.

3 A parting is made and the wrap is started by combing and directing away from the parting. At the same time, the other hand is used to smooth and blend the hair around the roller.

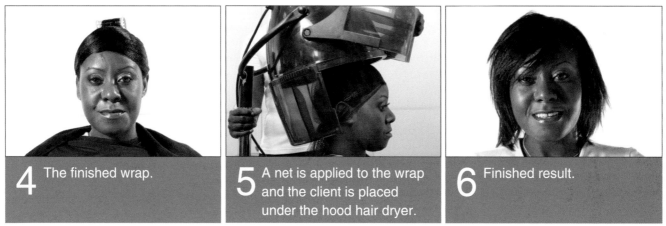

4 The finished wrap.

5 A net is applied to the wrap and the client is placed under the hood hair dryer.

6 Finished result.

HABIA AND CENGAGE LEARNING

IT'S A FACT!

The position of the roller at the crown is known as the 'point of origin'.

Making hair straight by blow drying (radial brush)

By using a large diameter radial brush, hair can be smoothed and straightened.

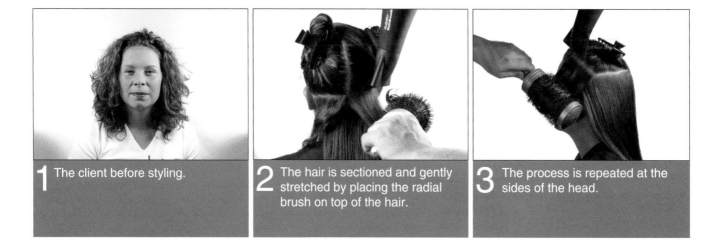

1 The client before styling.

2 The hair is sectioned and gently stretched by placing the radial brush on top of the hair.

3 The process is repeated at the sides of the head.

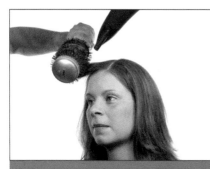

4 The process is completed at the front of the head. Note how smooth and straight the hair is.

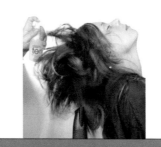

5 To create texture and movement the client tips their head back and cool air is blown into the hair from the dryer.

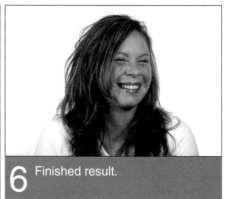

6 Finished result.

HABIA AND CENGAGE LEARNING

Making hair straight by blow drying and electrical equipment (paddle brush and straighteners)

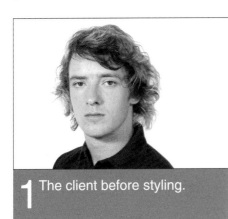

1 The client before styling.

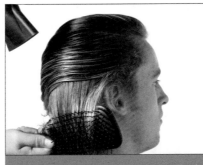

2 A styling product is applied and a paddle bush is used to smooth the hair.

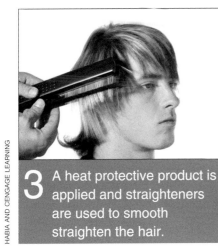

3 A heat protective product is applied and straighteners are used to smooth straighten the hair.

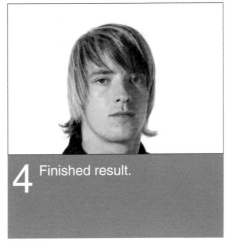

4 Finished result.

Making hair straight by using a rake attachment and thermal tongs

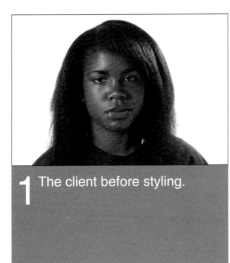

1 The client before styling.

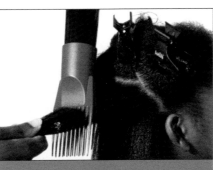

2 A rake attachment is used with a hand-held dryer. The rake is combed slowly through the hair, working from the ends to the roots.

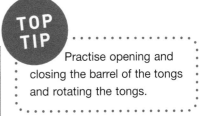

TOP TIP
Practise opening and closing the barrel of the tongs and rotating the tongs.

As pressing combs get very hot, you must check the temperature before applying it to the hair. To test, place the heated pressing comb on tissue. If the tissue becomes scorched, or burns, the comb is too hot and must be cooled by placing on a prepared cooling pad. The cooling pad is a pre-dampened, folded towel.

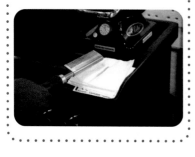

ACTIVITY

Work in pairs or on a mannequin head block and use techniques to straighten and smooth hair. Take a photograph of the end result. Identify what you did well and what you would do better next time.

SIGNPOST PLTS

PLTS

Creative thinker
Reflective learner
Teamworker
Self manager

You can make the hair curl by bending short hair over the finger while you are finger drying.

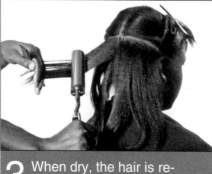

3 When dry, the hair is re-sectioned and thermal tongs are used to smooth and straighten the hair.

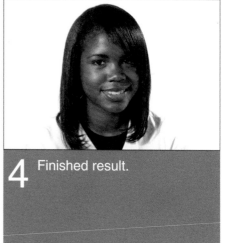

4 Finished result.

Other methods for making hair straight

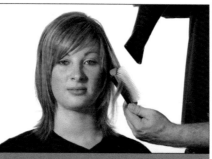

Hair can be smoothed using a flat back brush.

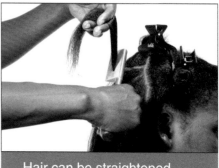

Hair can be straightened using a pressing comb.

Step-by-step method for finger drying hair

Finger drying is styling the hair using a hand-held hair dryer and your fingers. It is a very quick technique, but it only works well on short layered hair.

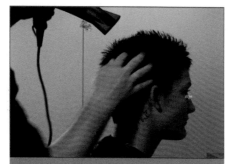

1 Following the shampoo, a styling product is applied to the hair. The fingers are used to hold the hair in place as the hair is dried.

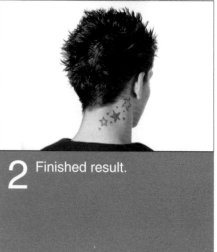

2 Finished result.

HABIA AND CENGAGE LEARNING

Step-by-step methods for plaiting and twisting hair

Creating one scalp plait

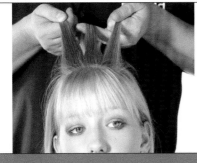

1 The first section is evenly divided into three stands.

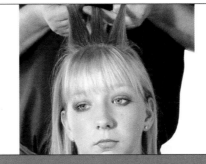

2 The strand on the right-hand side is passed over the centre strand.

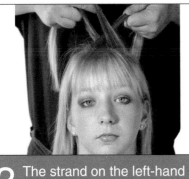

3 The strand on the left-hand side is passed over the centre strand.

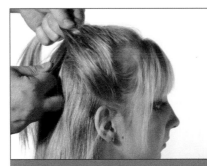

4 The process is repeated. Each time the outside strand is passed over the centre, hair is added to the strand from the hairline.

IT'S A FACT!

This type of scalp plait is usually called a *French plait*.

TOP TIP

When you are working at the back of the head, ask the client to bend their head forward to enable you to keep the plait close to the head.

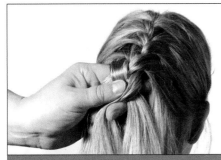

5 The plait continues down the back of the head. Be careful to keep the plait central and close to the head.

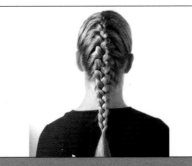

6 Finished result.

Creating multiple scalp plaits (corn row)

The same technique to create one plait is used to create multiple scalp plaits.

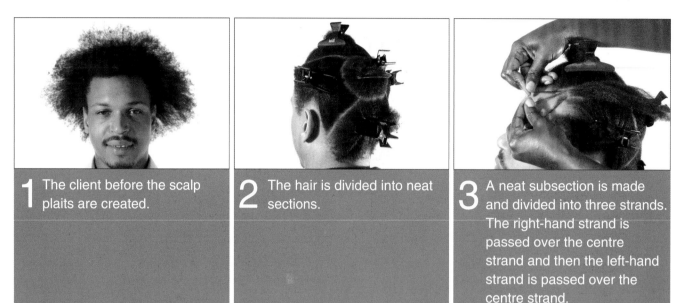

1 The client before the scalp plaits are created.

2 The hair is divided into neat sections.

3 A neat subsection is made and divided into three strands. The right-hand strand is passed over the centre strand and then the left-hand strand is passed over the centre strand.

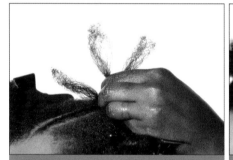

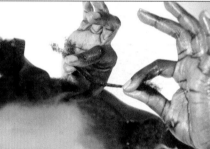

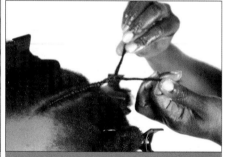

4 The process is repeated. Each time the outside strand is passed over the centre, hair is added to the strand from the outside of the section.

5 When the corn row is completed, divide the three strands into two.

6 Finish the corn row by twisting the two strands around each other.

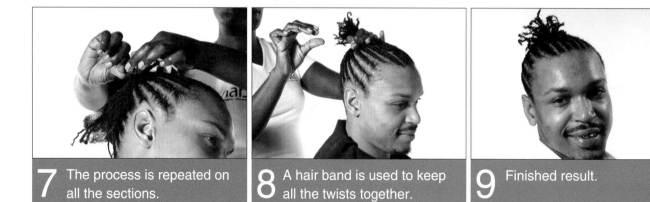

7 The process is repeated on all the sections.

8 A hair band is used to keep all the twists together.

9 Finished result.

Creating twists in hair

Scalp twists are similar to corn rows in that they are created using evenly spaced sections.

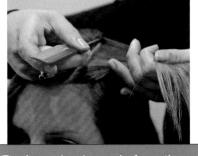

1 The client before the twists are created.

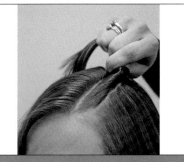

2 A section is made form the front hairline to the crown area.

3 Starting from the front hairline, the hair is twisted, following the pre-made section.

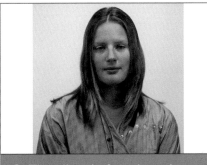

4 The twist is held in place with grips.

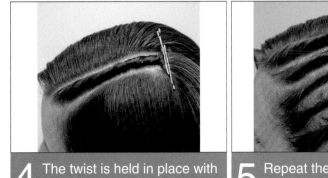

5 Repeat the process keeping the sections an even size.

TOP TIP

Do not pull the hair too tightly when making the twists as this can lead to increased tension at the roots.

ACTIVITY

Work in pairs or on a mannequin head block and use techniques to plait and twist hair. Take a photograph of the end result. Identify what you did well and what you would do better next time.

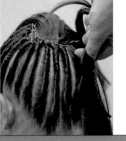

6 Repeat at the back of the head keeping the twists in place with hair grips.

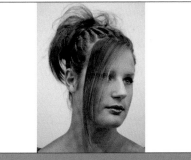

7 Finished result.

SIGNPOST PLTS

Creative thinker
Reflective learner
Teamworker
Self-manager

SIGNPOST PSD

Working towards goals

It takes a long time to master skills for styling, dressing, plaiting and twisting hair. The first time you try you may think that you will never be able to do it, but with practice you will see your skills improve all the time.

Work with your teacher to identify what you are really good at and what you need to improve. Set some goals that you would like to achieve over a few weeks or months. Write down the goals you would like to achieve. You may need some support to achieve them, so identify someone who can help you. Then review how you have done. Did you achieve your goals?

What you have learnt

The science behind hair styling

- Hair has properties of elasticity.

- The bonds in the cortex break temporarily so that you can change the shape of your hair.

- The hair can absorb moisture into itself from the atmosphere. This means that hair is hygroscopic.

- Your hairstyle will not last very long on humid and damp days because of the water vapour absorbed into the air from the atmosphere.

The factors that influence the choice of hair styles

- You must carry out a consultation with your client before you style their hair.

- Before you can begin to style hair, you must consider certain factors.

The tools, products and equipment you will use for plaiting, twisting, styling and dressing hair

- Tools must be sterilized before use on clients.

- All equipment should be made from materials that will not damage the hair.

- Electrical equipment should be used following the manufacturer's instructions and for the purpose for which it is intended.

- You must choose the correct product for hair type, texture and condition and for the purpose you are using it for.

How to prepare for plaiting, twisting, styling and dressing hair

- You must always be prepared when you are working with clients or helping others who are working with clients.

The basic techniques for plaiting, twisting, styling and dressing hair

- To create all hairstyles there are only four basic styling techniques. The techniques are:

  ○ Make hair look curly.

  ○ Make hair look wavy.

  ○ Make hair look straight.

  ○ Plait and twist hair.

ASSESSMENT ACTIVITIES

Activity 1 E1 – L1

How do you do that?

Look at the following hairstyles and then read the list of hairstyling techniques. Match the technique you would use to achieve the hairstyles.

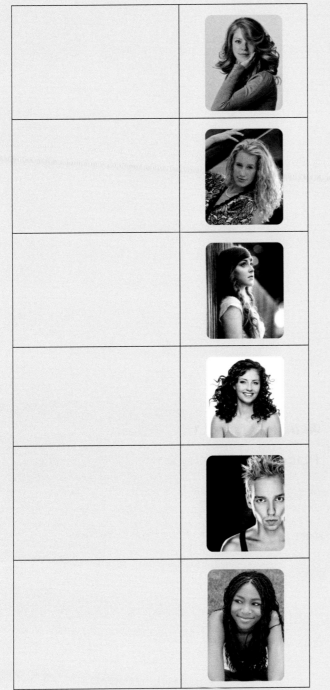

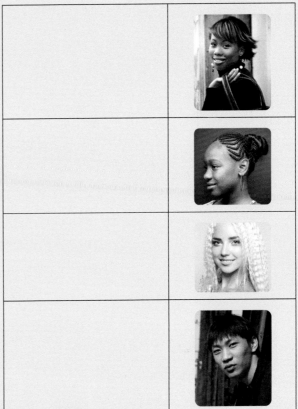

a. Blow dry and straighten.

b. Blow dry using a flat back brush.

c. Blow dry using a radial brush.

d. Crimp.

e. Curl using tongs.

f. Dry using a diffuser.

g. Finger dry.

h. Plait.

i. Scalp plait.

j. Set on heated rollers.

Activity 2 E3 – L1

Block Buster

Work with a partner or split into two teams. Choose a letter and answer the question. When you have answered the question correctly, mark off your square. See who can correctly answer the questions to complete a straight or diagonal line across the grid. You can block the way of your partner or other team to stop them winning!

B	C	R	T	P
E	W	F	R	G
S	A	P	D	W
T	O	B	T	S
F	C	P	C	T

B	Which Bs are broken when heat or water is used to style hair? _____
E	Which E is the property of hair that makes it able to stretch and return to its normal position? _____
S	Which S describes hair that is not curly? _____
T	Which T is the type of change to the hair structure during hair styling? _____
F	What are the Fs that you must consider before styling hair? _____
C	Which C is an example of hair texture? _____
W	Which W is an example of a hair type? _____
A	Which A is an example of hair density? _____
O	Which O is an example of a facial shape? _____
C	What C is the name of the process you carry out before you style your client's hair? _____
R	Which R is an example of a facial shape? _____
F	Which F is an example of hair texture? _____
P	Which P is the place on hair when you begin to de-tangle? _____

B	What are the Bs that you find on a hair brush? _____
P	Which P is a type of hair brush? _____
T	Which T is a type of comb? _____
R	What is the R that is used to curl hair? _____
D	What is the D that is used to dry hair without disturbing the natural curl? _____
T	Which T is used to store all your tools and equipment? _____
C	Which Cs are used to create tight wavy movements in hair? _____
P	What P is the name of the technique for weaving three strands of hair? _____
G	What is the G that is used to protect the client's clothes during hairstyling service? _____
W	What W is the name of a technique used to straighten hair? _____
S	What S is the electrical equipment that can be used to remove curl from hair? _____
T	What T is the electrical equipment that can be used to curl hair? _____

Activity 3 E1 – L1

Place the word

When you style your hair you are making a _____ change in the _____ of the hair. Because of this, your _____ does not last_____. The reason you can change the structure of your hair is because of some special_____ bonds in the _____ of the hair. They are special because they hold all the hair _____ together in its _____ position. So, if your hair is _____ curly, the bonds hold your hair in a curly position. If you hair is straight, the bonds will hold your hair in a naturally straight_____.

cortex	forever	natural	hairstyle	bonds
cells	naturally	position	temporary	structure

9

Safe and hygienic working practices

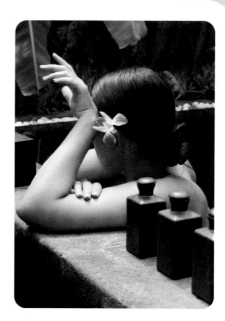

'Safety first' is 'Safety always'.

CHARLES M HAYES

In this chapter you will learn about:

- Safe and hygienic working practices.
- Sterilization and maintenance of tools and equipment.
- Awareness of the environment relating to the hair and beauty sector.
- Personal health and well-being.
- Correct posture.
- Healthy living and healthy lifestyle.

Introduction

We all need to work safely and hygienically, it helps protect us as individuals and also other people that come into contact with us. In this chapter you will be looking at different aspects of safe working practices that are needed in the hair and beauty sector. These will include the key parts of health and safety **legislation**, how you look after tools and equipment as well as your own personal conduct, well-being and safety.

Safe and hygienic working practices

Clients expect to see a clean and tidy salon. This means that during the day you will be expected to help make sure that the salon is kept clean, so that any client

IT'S A FACT!

When you are employed you will also be given a **job description** which will explain what you are expected to do in your job.

walking through the door will form a good first impression. This means that you will need to make sure that:

- Dirty cups and glasses are washed and put away.
- Floors and surfaces are kept clean and any hair, dirty materials or spillages removed straight away.
- Dirty towels and gowns are removed and stored ready for washing.
- Tools and equipment are cleaned, disinfected or sterilized before being used on another client.
- Used trolleys are cleaned and prepared ready for the next client.

It does not matter what position you have in the salon, everyone needs to take responsibility for health and safety. You have to take responsibility for how you behave and the actions you take. The salon will have a health and safety policy which will explain what everyone's responsibility is in the salon.

A clean hairdressing salon

TOP TIP

Always read work policies and procedures. They will provide the information needed to work safely in the salon.

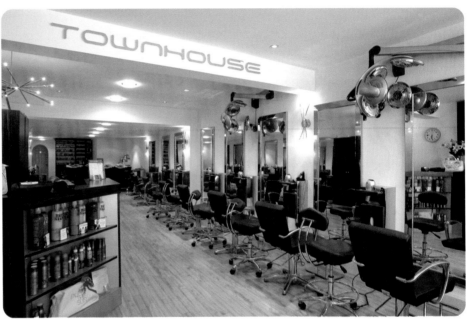

COURTESY OF REM

When working in a salon you need to be alert and aware of any potential hazards and risks that may cause an accident or hurt someone. If you can deal with the hazard you should do so quickly and safely. If you cannot deal with the problem yourself, you need to make sure you tell someone who can. This could be the person responsible for dealing with health and safety in the salon.

- A hazard is something with the potential to cause someone harm.
- A risk is the likelihood of someone's being harmed by the hazard.

For example, if a tap is leaking in the salon, it could be classed as a hazard. If that leaking tap was at the backwash area and there was a pool of water on the floor, someone could slip and hurt themselves. This would be a risk.

ACTIVITY

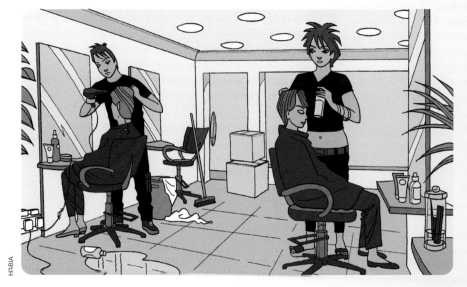

Spot the health and safety problems. List the health and safety issues that you have identified in the picture. Write down how you would deal with each issue.

SIGNPOST PLTS

Independent enquirer

English

When you write down how to deal with the health and safety issues, you will:

E3   write texts with some adaptation to the intended audience

L1   write a range of texts to communicate information, ideas and opinions, using formats and styles suitable for their purpose and intended audience.

SIGNPOST FUNCTIONAL SKILLS

Key health and safety legislation

There is legislation for all areas of safety when people are at work. The Health and Safety at Work Act (1974) is the main piece of legislation.

Health and safety legislation	Employer responsibility	Employee/trainee responsibility
Health and Safety at Work Act (1974)	Provide and maintain safety equipment and safe systems of work.	Not to interfere with or misuse anything provided for health and safety purposes, e.g. fire extinguishers.
	Make sure products and equipment are properly stored, handled and used.	Correctly use tools, products and equipment.

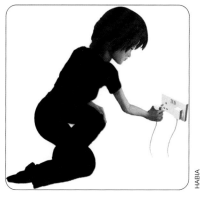

Trailing electrical flexes must be avoided

Health and safety legislation	Employer responsibility	Employee/trainee responsibility
	Provide information, training and supervision and make sure all employees are aware of and use manufacturer's instructions.	Use manufacturer's instructions.
	Provide a safe place to work and a safe environment.	Take care of their own health and safety.
	Look after the health and safety of clients.	Take care of the health and safety of team members and clients.
	Provide a written safety policy and carry out risk assessments.	Cooperate with the salon employer/manager.

IT'S A FACT!

The Health and Safety Executive (HSE) is the organization appointed by the government to support employers but also to make sure employers follow all health and safety laws and guidelines.

WHAT'S NEXT?

When you progress to Level 2 you will learn more about health and safety legislation for all aspects of working in a hair or beauty salon.

ACTIVITY

Find out about the types of personal protective equipment (PPE) that are used when carrying out different hair, beauty and nail services. Write a short report on your findings.

SIGNPOST PLTS

Independent enquirer

There is also legislation that covers:

- Procedures for when people at work have accidents or become ill.
- Procedures for employers to inform the Health and Safety Executive (HSE) of work-related accidents, diseases and dangerous occurrences.
- Employer's responsibility to maintain a safe, secure working environment.
- Employer's responsibility to provide suitable and safe equipment to be used at work.
- Employer's responsibility to provide **personal protective equipment** (PPE) that is to be used in the salon by employees.
- Procedures for using and storing chemicals, such as those that you will use in the hair and beauty sector.
- Requirements for employers to make sure all electrical equipment is checked by a qualified electrician.
- Procedures for the safe handling and manual lifting of heavy items.

SIGNPOST ERR

As part of employment rights and responsibilities when working in a salon means that you will need to show that you have a basic knowledge on issues relating to health and safety in the work place. This will include:

- Obeying all health and safety rules.
- Understanding how to use equipment and dangerous substances, in line with your training/instructions.
- How to conduct yourself in a safe manner.
- Understanding the correct method of waste disposal.

English

SIGNPOST
FUNCTIONAL
SKILLS

When you write about the personal protective equipment used in the hair and beauty industry, you will:

E3 write texts with some adaptation to the intended audience

L1 write a range of texts to communicate information, ideas and opinions, using formats and styles suitable for their purpose and audience.

TOP TIP

Make sure your posture is correct when lifting an object:

- Start with your hips, shoulders and feet in line.
- Centre the object to be lifted in front of you.
- Bend from the knees.
- Grasp the object firmly from underneath.
- Use your legs to lift the weight of the object.
- Make sure you are holding it comfortably.
- Carry the object walking upright.
- Remember to use your knees again when you put the object down.

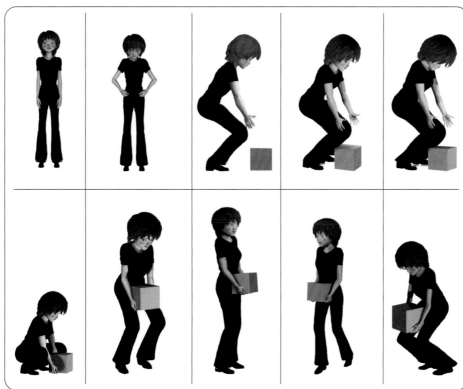

COURTESY OF L'OREAL/CENGAGE LEARNING

Safe lifting of boxes

ACTIVITY

You can find out more about health and safety from the Health and Safety Executive (HSE) website: **www.hse.gov.uk**

Once you have gathered information, design a leaflet, poster or mood board to present your ideas.

SIGNPOST
PLTS

Self-manager
Independent enquirer
Creative thinker
Reflective learner

ICT

SIGNPOST
FUNCTIONAL
SKILLS

When you are looking at websites for information from the HSE, you will interact with ICT for a given purpose and you will be able to recognize and use interface features. **E3** and **L1**.

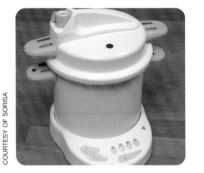

COURTESY OF SORISA

An autoclave

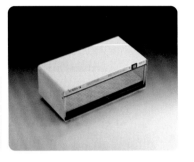

COURTESY OF SORISA

An ultraviolet lightbox

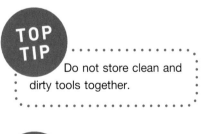

COURTESY OF SORISA

A Barbicide jar

TOP TIP
Do not store clean and dirty tools together.

TOP TIP
Always follow the manufacturer's instructions for cleaning and storing tools and equipment.

Sterilization and maintenance of tools and equipment

A professional stylist or therapist would never use dirty tools and equipment. How would you feel when you went to the hairdressers if the stylist brushed your hair with a hairbrush full of someone else's hair strands?

Different tools and equipment are cleaned, sterilized or disinfected in different ways.

There are three main methods of sterilising tools. These are:

- Heat: Use of an autoclave.
- Radiation: Use of an ultraviolet lightbox.
- Chemicals: Use of Barbicide.

Heat

Autoclaves are the most reliable method of sterilizing. They are used for sterilizing metal tools such as scissors, tweezers and cuticle nippers. They work by building up steam pressure and creating heat, which then destroys all living bacteria.

Radiation

A ultraviolet (UV) lightbox is often used in a salon for sterilizing tools such as brushes and combs. You must wash and dry the tools before putting them in the lightbox. The ultraviolet light uses **radiation** to prevent bacteria growth on the tools but complete **sterilization** is not guaranteed as the tools will only be sterilized on the areas where the UV rays reach. So it is important that the tools are turned over to make sure all areas have been exposed to the UV light.

Chemicals

Chemicals are the most commonly used method of disinfecting tools and equipment such as eyebrow tweezers and combs in the salon. In the hair and beauty sector a chemical called Barbicide is used. It is a clear blue low-level disinfectant. It does not sterilize tools but reduces the probability of infection. You must change Barbicide solution every day and the tools must be totally submerged in the solution and left in for the time recommended by the manufacturer.

Electrical tools and equipment cannot be sterilized or **disinfected** using the methods above. They must be wiped down to remove any debris or dirt before using them on a client.

Awareness of the environment relating to the hair and beauty sector

When working in the salon, there is also unused product and waste that needs to be disposed off. How we dispose of the different types of waste will depend on the local authority's policy.

Each local authority is responsible for **waste management**. Waste management is the collection, transport, processing and recycling or disposal of waste material. Wherever possible waste management will try to include environmental issues.

In the hair and beauty salon, the majority of waste produced is general waste some of which can be **recycled**.

However, salons can produce **clinical waste**. This type of waste must be kept apart from the general waste and disposed of separately by a licensed operator.

Clinical waste in the salon could include:

- Human tissue.
- Blood or other body fluids.
- Swabs, cotton wool or dressings.
- Syringes, blades or needles.

Other waste products such as perm lotion, colouring and lighting products can be disposed of by diluting them with water and pouring them down the sink.

When working in a salon, you want to work in a safe and pleasant **environment**. So not only is the correct and timely disposal of waste important but the atmosphere that we work in is also very important.

In Chapter 1, 'Understanding the hair and beauty sector', you will learn about the differences between hairdressing and beauty therapy salon environments.

Ventilation and temperature

No matter what type of salon you work in, it will need to have good **ventilation** and a comfortable temperature:

- Ventilation is important when dealing with chemicals that give off fumes or when carrying out nail extensions where lots of dust is created when filing the new nail.
- Temperature is important to make sure it is comfortable for everyone to work in but also for the client who may be sitting with wet hair or having a beauty treatment where they are in a state of undress.

IT'S A FACT!

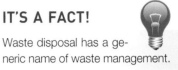

In the UK, around 330 million tonnes of waste is produced every year.

IT'S A FACT!

Waste disposal has a generic name of waste management.

IT'S A FACT!

Recycling involves extracting and reprocessing waste into new products.

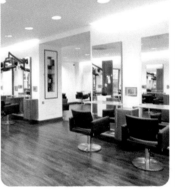

HOBBS SALONS, TEMPLE FORTUNE, LONDON

A hairdressing salon

A beauty therapy room

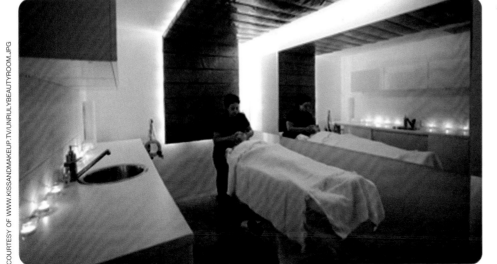

COURTESY OF WWW.KISSANDMAKEUP.TV/UNRULYBEAUTYROOM.JPG

Hot water, heat and electricity

Hot water, heat and electricity are used in all hair and beauty salons. Without these three main facilities you would not be able to deliver treatments or services to your clients.

Water

Water is very important, without it you would not be able to function in the salon. It is used for everything from cleaning the salon to washing client's hair as well as washing your hands.

There are two types of water, hard and soft:

- Hard water contains a quantity of dissolved minerals.
- Soft water contains fewer quantities of dissolved minerals.

Hard water is not as user friendly as soft water. It may shorten the life of equipment and does not help products such as shampoo to lather and perform as well as they would do with soft water.

Heat

In some beauty treatments, heat can be beneficial to pre-heat the body's muscles prior to or as part of the treatment. It helps to relax the muscles and make

A steamer and accelerator

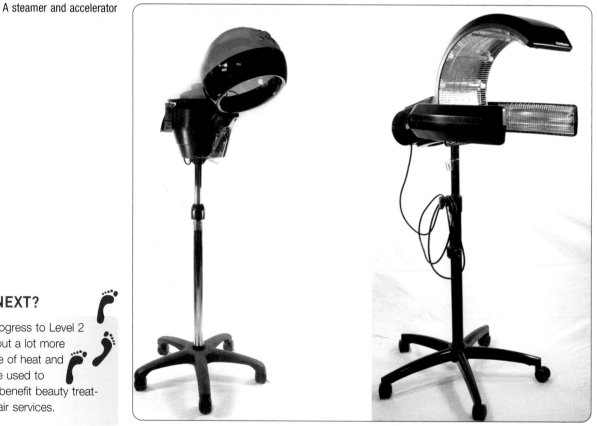

WHAT'S NEXT?

When you progress to Level 2 you will find out a lot more about the use of heat and how it can be used to support and benefit beauty treatments and hair services.

HABIA

the treatment more effective. Heat is often used in the form of saunas, steam rooms, showers or Jacuzzis as part of spa treatments.

In hair services, warm water helps the hair cuticle to soften and open to allow the penetration of products. Equipment such as steamers can be used to open up the cuticle or heat can be used to reduce the development time of colour services. Heat is also used to soften the hair structure to allow you to change its shape; you do this when you blow dry the hair or use electrically heated equipment.

Electricity

Electricity provides power for the lights in the salon and the technical equipment that you use to carry out treatments or services. It is also needed at the reception desk if the salon uses computerized appointment and payment systems.

Could you imagine life without these three important utilities?

ACTIVITY

List the different types of electrical equipment that can be used in the hair or beauty salon. What are they used for?

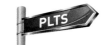

SIGNPOST PLTS

Independent enquirer

SIGNPOST FUNCTIONAL SKILLS

ICT

If you use a computer to design a table explaining what the electrical equipment is used for, you will:

use ICT to develop, present and communicate information at **E3** and **L1**.

Personal health and well-being

In Chapter 2, you learnt about the importance of personal hygiene. How washing your hands correctly and regularly will minimize the risk of cross infection. Washing hands during a treatment also illustrates to your client that you have a hygienic and professional attitude.

Looking after yourself is also very important, so that you do not become ill or injured. Working in the hair and beauty industries is a tiring job. It is important that you are aware of how to work safely to protect your health so that you can have a long and exciting future in the world of hair and beauty. To protect yourself you must always be aware of the dangers and how to avoid them. Employers should have work policies and procedures to explain how to carry out your job safely. They will provide personal protective equipment (PPE) that you should always use. Manufacturers will also provide instructions of how to use and prepare products and equipment safely.

Always work sensibly and responsibly to protect yourself.

There are a number of health areas that you need to be aware of as they can affect people working in the hair and beauty sector. These are:

- Repetitive strain injury (RSI): Term used to describe symptoms that occur when you have carried out a repetitive task such as holding a hairdryer or turning hairbrushes for long periods of time.

- Asthma: Term given to a condition where a person's airways become irritated and inflamed. They become narrow and produce extra mucus. The type of asthma that you can be affected by in the salon is called

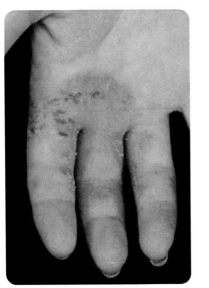

Contact dermatitis

occupational asthma. Occupational asthma is caused by chemical products or fine particles of dust. That is why it is important that the salon environment has a good ventilation system to remove them. But it is important that you wear PPE, including wearing a dust mask when mixing powder-based products.

● Skin sensitivity: Term used when the skin reacts to a substance, creating redness, spots or pustules and skin erosion. Sensitive skin tends to be irritated by many common items, such as chemicals found in fragrances, lanolin which can be found in cosmetic products and alkalis in detergents and shampoos.

● Dermatitis is a common form of skin sensitivity and contact dermatitis is a condition that can affect people working in hair and beauty salons. Contact dermatitis is an itchy skin condition caused by an allergic reaction to certain materials. Products such as shampoos that you are in constant contact with can cause irritation. It is important that after shampooing hair you wash and dry your hands and apply a good hand cream to protect them. To help prevent contact dermatitis always wear protective, disposable, non-latex gloves to protect your hands from water and chemicals.

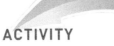

SIGNPOST
PLTS

Independent enquirer

ACTIVITY

Why not find out more about looking after your hands? You can research this information from the Habia health and safety website **www.habia.org/healthandsafety/** you will find video clips on how to wash your hands and how to wear and remove gloves correctly.

SIGNPOST
FUNCTIONAL
SKILLS

ICT

When you are looking at websites for information on health and safety, you will interact with ICT for a given purpose and you will be able to recognize and use interface features. **E3** and **L1**

WHAT'S NEXT?

When progressing to Level 2 hairdressing or beauty therapy you will learn more about looking after your health and well-being. You will also learn about the importance of using personal protective equipment (PPE) and how to safeguard against occupational injury.

Correct posture

Most of us are concerned with our health but very few of us pay attention to our **posture**.

Making sure that your posture is correct will help your long-term health and well-being. It will help you have a longer career in the hair and beauty sector by preventing occupational injuries and it will also make you look and feel more confident.

Like all hair and beauty professionals, you will need to learn how to have good posture to ensure that your stance is even and you have good body balance as

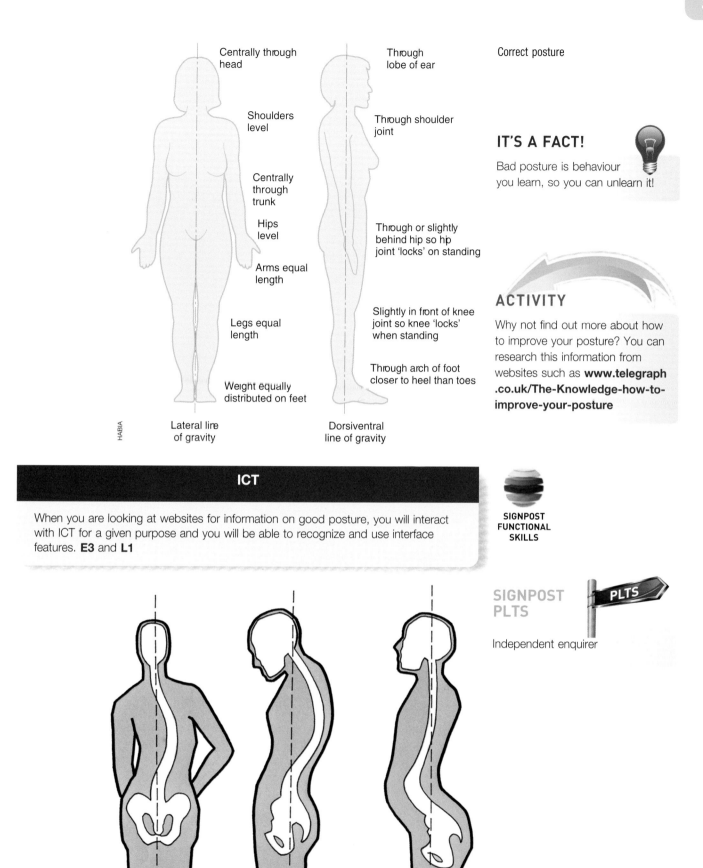

Centrally through head

Shoulders level

Centrally through trunk

Hips level

Arms equal length

Legs equal length

Weight equally distributed on feet

Lateral line of gravity

Through lobe of ear

Through shoulder joint

Through or slightly behind hip so hip joint 'locks' on standing

Slightly in front of knee joint so knee 'locks' when standing

Through arch of foot closer to heel than toes

Dorsiventral line of gravity

Correct posture

HABIA

IT'S A FACT!

Bad posture is behaviour you learn, so you can unlearn it!

ACTIVITY

Why not find out more about how to improve your posture? You can research this information from websites such as **www.telegraph .co.uk/The-Knowledge-how-to-improve-your-posture**

ICT

When you are looking at websites for information on good posture, you will interact with ICT for a given purpose and you will be able to recognize and use interface features. **E3** and **L1**

SIGNPOST FUNCTIONAL SKILLS

SIGNPOST PLTS

PLTS

Independent enquirer

Posture faults

HABIA

ACTIVITY

Practice standing so that you have the correct posture. How does it feel? Is it very different from how you normally stand?

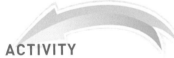

SIGNPOST
PLTS

Self-manager

ACTIVITY

In a group, discuss how drinking alcohol or taking drugs can affect a person's health and personality.

SIGNPOST
PLTS

Teamwork
Effective participators

you work around the salon and your clients. So that you can work at the correct height and to maintain your body balance while working, the height of some stools or chairs can be adjusted. Standing and sitting with the proper postural alignment will help you work more effectively, creating less strain on your body.

Good posture is achieved when your head, shoulders, upper torso and abdomen, thighs and legs distribute your body's weight evenly over your feet. Your feet should be faced forward and slightly apart. If you move position and lower one of your hips, it will change the balance of your body and put extra weight on that leg and foot. It will cause your spine to curve and put strain and discomfort on the lower part of your back.

How to check your posture:

● Stand with the back of your head touching the wall.

● Your heels should be 150 mm from the wall.

● Your bottom should touch the wall.

● Check the distance with your hand between your neck and the wall. If you are within 50 mm at the neck, you have pretty good posture.

Healthy living and healthy lifestyle

Becoming a professional stylist, therapist or technician is all about looking after your clients and the treatments and services you will be carrying out. It can be very hard work that is both physically and mentally demanding:

● Physically, you are on your feet all day, holding and moving equipment and stretching and using different parts of your body to carry out some of the treatments or services.

● Mentally, you listen to, talk, advise and make decisions with and for your clients.

Being prepared for work in a salon is about how you act, the choices and decisions you make and how you live your life, the food you eat and how you look after your health. These will all affect how well you carry out your job.

You need to be fit and healthy to meet the demands of the job.

Eating a **balanced diet** and regular exercise is very important to healthy living. Getting enough sleep during the week when you are working will enable you to work more effectively.

Understanding how drinking alcohol or using drugs will have an effect on your body and how they can affect your behaviour is very important, particularly when you are working with people all day at work.

This does not mean that you cannot enjoy yourself. It is about making sure that you can give your best at work and have energy to enjoy yourself outside work. It is about getting the right work–life balance.

English

When you have your discussion, you will:

E3 respond appropriately to others and make some extended contributions in familiar formal and informal discussions and exchanges

L1 take part in formal and informal discussions and exchanges that include unfamiliar subjects.

SIGNPOST FUNCTIONAL SKILLS

Your overall health is reflected in your skin. If you feel under the weather or have been ill for some time, then your skin will suffer. The skin needs to have a good blood supply bringing oxygen and **nutrients** to every cell. Anything that disrupts this process will have an effect on the health and appearance of your skin.

It is therefore important that you eat healthily, drink lots of water and get regular exercise.

Fresh air is also very good for you and your skin.

A balanced diet containing vitamins such as vitamin C will help improve skin healing and vitamin E will help improve the skin's condition.

Healthy eating

A good diet is central to your overall good health. A balanced diet is not about banning or leaving out any type of food but balancing what you eat by eating a variety of foods from each of the different food groups in the right amounts.

Eat different types of food to make sure you get all the essential nutrients.

TOP TIP

The five-a-day rule recommends that to stay healthy we should eat five servings of fruit and vegetables every day. One serving can include items such as:

- One medium sized apple.

- Half a cup of beans, chopped fruit or vegetables.

- A cup of leafy salad leaves or a small glass of fresh fruit juice.

IT'S A FACT!

Potatoes do not count as one of your five-a-day because they are made up of starches.

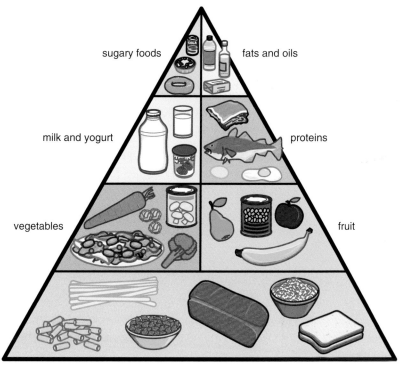

Balanced diet

A balanced diet

Food type	What it does	Which food you can find them in
Carbohydrates	Give you energy.	Found in potatoes, rice, pasta, bread and cereals.
Proteins	Enable you to grow and repair your body and give you energy.	Found in red and white meat, fish, eggs, cheese and milk.
Fats	Used as a form of energy. Unsaturated fats help your heart stay healthy.	Found in fish such as tuna and salmon, olive oil and peanut oil.
Vitamins	Vitamin A is good for your eyes. Vitamin B is good for the immune and nervous system. There are different types of vitamin B. Vitamin C helps the body repair itself. Vitamin D is good for the absorption of calcium. Vitamin E helps in reproduction.	Found in meat, vegetables, fruit, fish, nuts, rice, pasta, eggs and butter.
Mineral salts	Iron is needed to make haemoglobin in our blood. Calcium is needed to give us strong healthy teeth, bones and muscles. Sodium is used by all your cells especially the nervous system.	Found in fish, meat, milk, seeds, nuts, fruit, vegetables and salt.
Fibre	Used to help your digestive system work properly.	Found in fruit, vegetables, nuts, seeds and pulses along with rice and wholemeal or granary bread.

Fruit and vegetables should make up about one-third of your daily diet and can be eaten as part of every meal. You should eat five portions of fruit and vegetables each day.

Bread, rice, potatoes and pasta should also make up one-third of your diet as they contain the starchy carbohydrates that give your body its main source of energy. Wholegrain foods are rich in fibre and other nutrients that have many health benefits.

The final third of your daily food intake should be made up of food that needs to be eaten in smaller proportions. They are still needed for our balanced diet so it is important that you do not leave them out:

- Milk and dairy foods should be eaten in moderation because they have a high saturated fat content, but they are an important source of calcium.

- Meat, fish, eggs and beans are a source of animal and plant protein. This form of protein gives us energy and is needed for growth and repair.

- Food and drinks that are high in fat or sugar should make up the smallest part of your daily intake. They should only be eaten in small amounts because they contain very few nutrients and are high in unhealthy components, such as saturated fats and sugar or salt, that are associated with increasing the risks to your health.

ACTIVITY

Nutrition and exercise is important to a healthy life. Make a record of the food you eat each day for a week and the exercise that you take:

● Can you identify the different food groups that you have eaten?

● Is it a balanced diet?

● If not, what simple changes can you make to your diet?

● Do you think you do enough exercise?

Design a chart or mood board of the food you would like to eat that would give you a balanced diet. Also include the type of exercise that you would do to help keep you healthy and fit.

You can then present your chart to your team.

ACTIVITY

Why not find out more about a balanced diet? You can research information from the Food Standards Agency website **www.eat-well.gov.uk**

SIGNPOST PLTS

Independent enquirer
Self-manager
Reflective learner
Effective participator
Creative thinker

SIGNPOST FUNCTIONAL SKILLS

English
When you write about the food you have eaten and tell others about it, you will:

E3 write texts with some adaptation to the intended audience

L1 write a range of texts to communicate information, ideas and opinions, using formats and styles suitable for their purpose and audience

E3 respond appropriately to others and make some extended contributions in familiar formal and informal discussions and exchanges

L1 take part in formal and informal discussions and exchanges that include unfamiliar subjects.

SIGNPOST FUNCTIONAL SKILLS

ICT
When you are looking at websites for information from the Food Standards Agency, you will interact with ICT for a given purpose and you will be able to recognize and use interface features. **E3** and **L1**

You will also use developing, presenting and communicating information at **E3** and **L1** if you develop a chart or any presentation material using ICT.

What you have learnt

● Safe and hygienic working practices:

　○ The importance of a clean and tidy salon.

● Sterilization and maintenance of tools and equipment.

● Awareness of the environment relating to the hair and beauty sector:

○ The importance of ventilation and temperature.

○ How salons use electricity, water and heat.

● Personal health and well-being:

● Correct posture:

○ Why it is important to have good posture.

● Healthy living and healthy lifestyle:

○ The importance of healthy eating.

ASSESSMENT ACTIVITY

Activity 1 L1

Short answer questions:

1   Explain the difference between a hazard and a risk.

2   Name three hazards that you could find in the salon.

3   What does PPE stand for?

4   Name two items of PPE.

5   Who is responsible for checking the condition of electrical equipment?

Activity 2 E3 and L1

Food groups

Identify the type of food in the left-hand column and write down in the right-hand column the food group that it supplies.

TYPE OF FOOD	FOOD GROUP

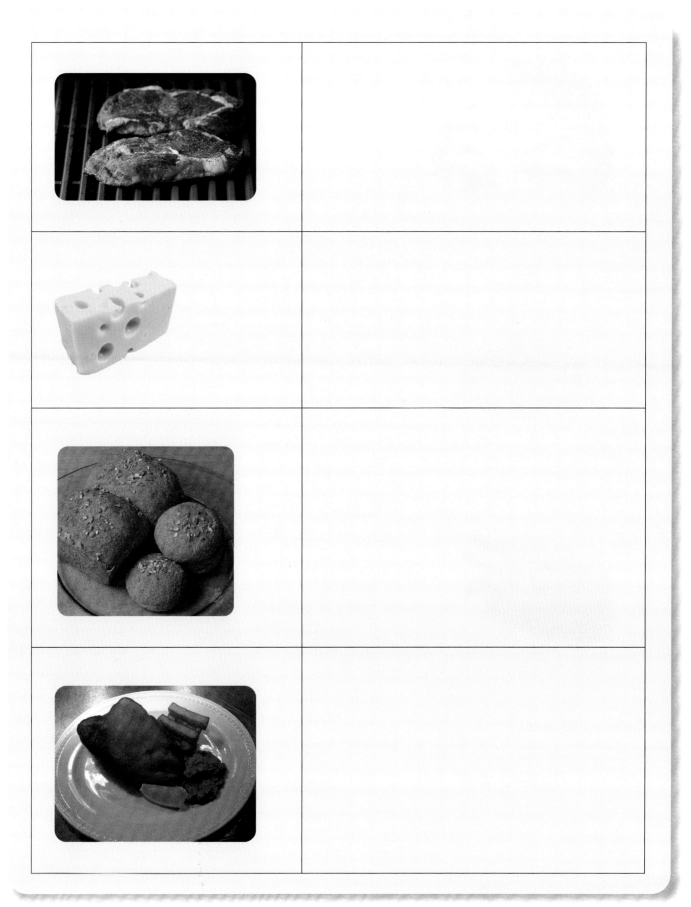

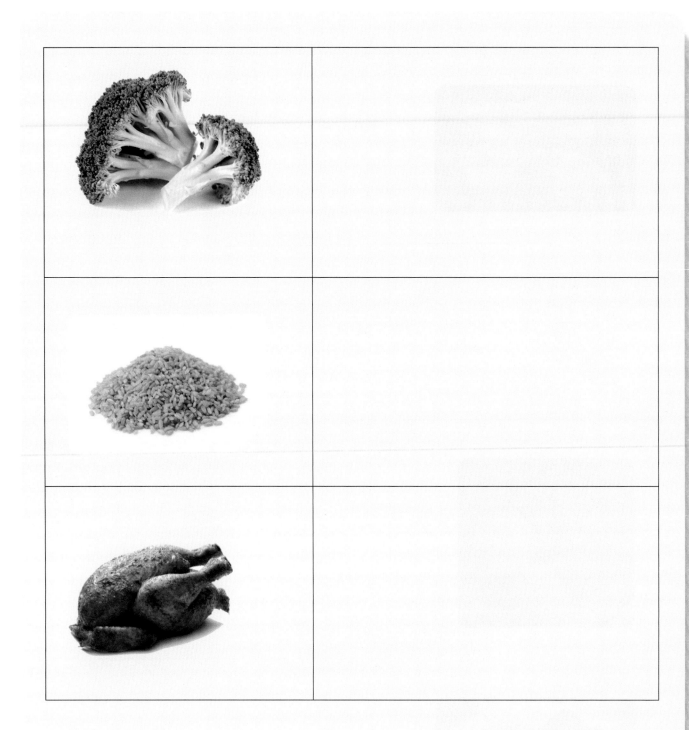

Activity 3E3 and L1

Healthy living and healthy lifestyle

Complete the following text by adding the correct word/s from the table into the missing spaces:

beauty therapist	healthy	skin	diet	behaviour
exercise	choices	water	oxygen	vitamin
alcohol	energy	mentally	hormonal	sleep

Becoming a professional stylist, therapist or _____ is all about looking after your clients and the treatments and services you will be carrying out. It can be very hard work that is both physically and mentally demanding.

- Physically, you are on your feet all day, holding and moving equipment and stretching and using different parts of your body to carry out some of the treatments or services.

- _____, you listen to, talk, advise and make decisions with and for your clients.

Being prepared for work in a salon is about how you act, the _____ and decisions you make and about how you live your life, the food you eat and the way you look after your health. These will all affect how well you carry out your job.

You need to be fit and _____ to meet the demands of the job.

Eating a balanced diet and regular _____ is very important to healthy living. Getting enough _____ during the week when you are working will enable you to work more effectively.

Understanding how drinking _____ or using drugs will have an effect on your body and how they can affect your _____ is very important, particularly when you are working with people all day at work.

This does not mean that you cannot enjoy yourself. It is about making sure that you can give your best at work and have _____ to enjoy yourself outside work. It is about getting the right work–life balance.

Your overall health is reflected in your skin. If you feel under the weather or have been ill for some time, then your skin will suffer. The _____ needs to have a good blood supply bringing _____ and nutrients to every cell. Anything that disrupts this process will have an effect on the health and appearance of your skin.

It is therefore important that you eat healthily, drink lots of _____ and get regular exercise.

Fresh air is also very good for you and your skin.

A balanced _____ containing vitamins such as _____ C will help improve skin healing and vitamin E will help improve the skin's condition.

Some people feel that the face can reflect problems elsewhere in the body, for example:

- A breakout of spots on your chin could be linked to constipation.

- Spots under your jaw at either side of your face could be linked to a _____ imbalance.

Glossary

Abbreviations A shortened form of a word or words.

Abundant A description for the amount of hair on the head, abundant being lots of hair.

Accurately To do something carefully or precisely.

Acid mantle The protective coating on the skin's surface that helps protect it from bacteria.

Airbrushing The process of applying make-up using an airbrush. The airbrush turns the liquid make-up into a fine mist.

Allergic reaction A reaction to make-up which may result in redness, swelling or irritation.

Anagen, catagen and telogen The names of the different stages of the hair growth cycle.

Antiseptic A sanitizer, suitable for use on the skin.

Appointment An arrangement to meet at a set time and place.

Apprentice A person undergoing a formal training programme in a particular industry. The training programme is called an apprenticeship.

Apprenticeship An employer training programme.

Apprenticeship framework The requirements and different qualifications that are needed to complete an apprenticeship.

Arrector pili The muscle attached to the hair that makes the hair stand on end when you are cold or frightened.

Astringent A strong form of skin toner used on oily skin.

Balanced diet Appropriate proportions of different food types to keep you healthy.

Body odour Unpleasant smell of stale sweat, dirt and bacteria.

Brief A description outlining the requirements for a project.

Budget plan A system of recording the amount of money you are spending against the money that you have available to spend.

Camouflage make-up Make-up to minimize unwanted skin tones or skin blemishes.

Chromotherapy Spa and beauty treatments using colours to soothe, relax, energize.

Client A customer who pays money for hairdressing or beauty services.

Clinical waste Waste that contains human tissue such as blood or body fluid.

Colour spectrum All the individual colours that separate from white light.

Commission A percentage of the money paid by clients for the treatments and services that are carried out that is given to the stylist or therapist as part of their wage.

Complementary colours Colours that are opposite each other on a colour circle.

Consultation Examination of and communication with a client prior to a service or treatment.

Contact dermatitis A skin condition usually found on the hands and arms following a reaction to products and chemicals.

Contract of employment A legal agreement between an employer and employee which states the conditions of employment.

Cortex The inner section of hair.

Cranium Eight bones that protect the brain.

Credit card When someone pays using a credit card, the amount is not taken from the bank account immediately; they receive a monthly bill for all the transactions they have made in that period.

Cross-infection Transfer of infection, from one area of the body to another or to another person.

Cuticle Layer of dead tissue around the edge of the nail plate that seals the space between the skin and the nail plate. The term cuticle is also used to describe the outer layer of each individual hair strand.

Debit card Card issued by the bank to allow the transaction of payment or the withdrawal of money from your account.

Depth How light or how dark the hair is e.g., light brown, dark blonde, black.

Dermis The inner layer of the skin, just under the epidermis.

Disinfecting Removing germs such as bacteria.

Double dip Dipping a make-up applicator into a container after using on the skin of the client.

Elasticity Hair in good condition has the ability to stretch and return to its normal length.

Elasticity test A test used to check the condition of the inner layer of the hair, the cortex.

Employability skills The skills required to succeed in employment.

Environment The physical surroundings and general conditions that are around us.

Epidermis The outer layer of the skin.

Formal An agreed process, procedure or look.

Free edge Section of the nail plate that extends beyond the finger.

Hair growth cycle The continuous pattern of hair growth and hair loss.

Hair growth patterns The different directions for hair growth usually found at the nape of the neck, the crown area and the front hairline.

Harmonious colours Colours that are next to each other on a colour circle.

High definition A high-quality image used in television and film.

Holistic therapies Therapies that treat the individual as a whole – treating the mind, the body and the spirit.

Hygiene Set of practices and procedures to protect the health of you and others.

Hygroscopic Hair has the ability to draw water vapour into itself.

Job description A list of procedures and activities that a person has been employed to do.

Keratin The protein in the skin that makes it tough and prevents substances passing through it.

Leave-in conditioners A conditioner applied and left in the hair.

Legislation Laws and regulations.

Lunula Part of the nail matrix that can be seen at the base of the nail; also called the half moon.

Lymphatic A system that helps remove waste products such as urea and toxins from the body.

Manicure A treatment that involves the care of the hands and fingernails.

Melanin A pigment found in hair and skin which determines the colour of the hair or skin.

Micro-organisms Very tiny organisms that cannot be seen with the naked eye, including bacteria, fungi and viruses.

Mood board A collection of items that are gathered together, based on a theme.

Nerves Fibres or bundles of fibres carrying impulses/messages between the brain and other areas of the body.

Nodules Small round lumps in the muscles caused by a build-up of tension, tightness or swelling.

Non-verbal communication Using body language to transmit our feelings to someone, such as hand gestures or smiling.

Nutrients Substances that provides essential foods for the maintenance of life.

Occupational asthma Caused by chemical products or fine particles of dust from skin and nails.

Pay slip The record of the amount you are paid and the deductions that have been taken for tax purposes.

Pedicure A treatment that involves the care of the feet and toenails.

Personal conduct How a person behaves, the actions and words you use in different situations.

Personal protective equipment (PPE) Equipment used to protect you from harmful chemicals or particles.

Physical communication Method of communication involving physical contact, i.e. touching.

Porosity test A test used to check the condition of the outside layer of the hair, the cuticle.

Positive impression How we decide that something is good from the information we take in from hearing, seeing and touching.

Posture Position of the body.

Preparation for work qualification A qualification that leads to skills and knowledge required to prepare you for employment.

Primary colours of light Red, blue and green.

Primary colours of pigment Red, yellow and blue.

Puberty The period of time at which adolescents reach sexual maturity and become capable of having children.

Radiation Heat is transmitted without contact.

Recycling Reprocessing waste into new products.

Sebaceous gland The gland that produces sebum.

Sebum Natural oily substance found on the skin.

Sector The general term that is used to describe all the separate industries found in hair and beauty.

Services The name given to the different things that clients have done at the hairdressers such as a haircut or a hair colour.

Skull The bones that make up the cranium and the face.

Smoky eyes An eye make-up application using darker colours such as black, dark grey and dark brown on the edges of the upper and lower eyelids which are blended over the eyelid.

Sparse A description for the amount of hair on the head, sparse being very little hair.

Sterilization To totally destroy any micro-organisms on tools or equipment.

Subcutaneous layer This layer separates the dermis from the muscles. It is a storage area for fat.

Suture The joining that fuses the cranium bones together to form the skull.

Symmetrical Two structures or objects that have equal shape and size and similar position. A repetition of exactly the same parts.

Teamwork Working together to get the best result.

Terminal hair Hair found on the head or in the beard.

Tertiary colours Colours made from secondary colours.

Tone The colour that you see in hair e.g., red, copper, golden.

Toner A hairdressing colour product used to subdue unwanted tones in hair or enhance the natural colour of hair.

Traction alopecia A hair loss condition caused by excessive tension on the hair roots.

Treatments The name given to the different things that clients have done at the beauty salon such as a facial or a manicure.

Trial run A practice session used prior to the actual event.

Vellus hair Soft, fine and downy hair.

Ventilation Causes air to circulate around the room.

Verbal communication Method of communication such as speaking.

Visual aids Examples are style books which are used to help clients choose a new look for hair, make-up or nail art.

Waste management Collection, transport, processing, recycling or otherwise disposing of waste.

Well-being A term commonly used to describe what is good for a person, especially when it is related to a person's health.

Work-based learning Learning through employment.

Work policies Set of formal written procedures for employees to follow.

Work-ready qualification A qualification that leads to skills and knowledge required for employment.

Zinc pyrithione or selenium sulphide Ingredients found in shampoos used to treat dandruff.

Index